PHYSICAL

Farrar, Straus and Giroux

New York

PHYSICAL

An American Checkup

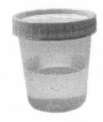

JAMES McMANUS

FARRAR, STRAUS AND GIROUX
19 Union Square West, New York 10003

Grateful acknowledgment is made to the following for permission to reprint previously published material:
Excerpt from "Tobacco," by Graham Lee Hemminger, is reprinted by permission of the Penn State University Archives, Pennsylvania State University Libraries.
"Church, State Joyfully Reunite After 230-Year Trial Separation" is reprinted with permission of *The Onion*. Copyright 2003 by Onion, Inc. www.theonion.com.
Excerpt from "Reagan's Next Victory," by William Safire, copyright © 2004 by The New York Times Co. Reprinted with permission.

Library of Congress Cataloging-in-Publication Data
McManus, James.
        Physical : an American checkup / James McManus.— 1st ed.
            p.   cm.
        ISBN-13: 978-0-374-23202-3 (hardcover : alk. paper)
        ISBN-10: 0-374-23202-4 (hardcover : alk. paper)
            1. McManus, James—Health. 2. Social medicine—United States.
        3. Medical care—United States. 4. Middle-aged persons—Health
        and hygiene—United States—Case studies.   I. Title.

    RA418.3.U6M36 2006
    362.1'0973—dc22

                                                            2005018726

Designed by Gretchen Achilles

Title page photograph by Samantha Cosentino

www.fsgbooks.com

1   3   5   7   9   10   8   6   4   2

For my girls—
Bridget, Jennifer, Beatrice, Grace

I must study the plain, physical facts of the case, ascertain what is possible, and learn what appears to be wise and right.

—ABRAHAM LINCOLN

CONTENTS

PHYSICAL

THAT'S THAT

I looked away to the hills
Above the river, where the golden lights of sunset

And sunrise are one and the same, and I saw something flying
Back and forth, fluttering its wings. Then it stopped in mid-air.
It was an angel, one of the good ones, about to sing.

—MARK STRAND, *Dark Harbor, XLV*

I would kiss the diamondback if I knew it would get me to heaven.

—LUCINDA WILLIAMS, "Get Right with God"

The truth is, I don't think I'm going to die. Not today, not tomorrow, not in 2067. Not me. To begin with, I'm careful and lucky enough not to get hit by a bus. An SUV maybe, or the culture of SUVs, or the cult—but no bus. I'm also immune by dint of heredity to most forms of cancer, by passport to snakebite and tropical maladies, by suburb and commuting pattern to Al Qaeda, by neck of the woods to tsunamis and hurricanes and earthquakes and floods, and by basic straight wholesome good old-fashioned solid moral American core family values (or at least a fear of needles) to overdose and sexually transmitted diseases. I'm bulletproof. At the same time, I try pretty hard never to imagine those eight hyphenated integers after my name or under my black-and-white photograph. No, not my zip code or social security number—those both have nine. Phone number? Ten. I'm talking 1951–20whatever.

Right now I'm fifty-four, a baby boomer gone mostly gray on the top and squishier than I'd like through the middle. I'm no Orson Welles or Chris Farley, no late Brando or early Belushi, but the small of my back, well, it isn't so small anymore. Otherwise I seem to be in reasonably half-decent shape for a fellow my age. Plus I'm bulletproof, baby! So it doesn't really matter, you see, that my father had his first heart attack at forty-six and a fatal stroke at sixty-one. Or that *his* father, the man for whom I was named, died of a heart attack at thirty-five, when my father was seven months old. Or that my kid brother Kevin, who was named for our father, died at forty-one of complications after a marrow transplant at Johns Hopkins, the best leukemia treatment center on the planet. A funny, athletic, warmhearted guy who wrote features for *The Washington Post*, he was in such bionic shape that it took a couple of weeks for even total renal failure to kill him, and his wife and mother and siblings got to watch every minute. "How'm I doin'?" he gasped upon briefly emerging, blind and desperate, from his final coma. "How're the kids?" My doubles partner, an ophthalmological surgeon, developed frontal lobe dementia and doesn't recognize his wife and children anymore, let alone me; needless to say, he no longer plays tennis or practices medicine. My caustically hilarious editor at Harper-Collins died in 2001 after a long illness. The woman who taught me how to play poker died on her ninetieth birthday. On his way in through a Wrigley Field turnstile in September 2004, my of-

4

fice mate and fellow geezer dad's hyper, magnificent brain was drowned in its own blood by an aneurysm. In 1999 my fourth child (third daughter) made an unexpected footling breech presentation, got her neck lodged between her mother's abdominal muscles during the C-section, and almost snapped her spine or strangled herself getting born. Two years later my son, a scorchingly talented guitarist who was named after me—me, who has less than zero musical talent—died of a drug overdose in a mental health clinic at age twenty-two. Suicide? It would not have been the first time he tried. Medication mistake by a nurse? Autopsy report inconclusive; lawsuit pending. At least two pharmaceutical companies who made antidepressants prescribed for him, Wyeth and GlaxoSmithKline, had lied about data suggesting links between their drugs and suicide in teenagers; lawsuits pending. Not that legal maneuvers or money can bring James back to us, or retroactively soothe all the pain he was in. Executing by hand the persons who manipulated the data and made the decisions to keep pushing those antidepressants wouldn't accomplish that, either, though I'd still love to do it. In any event, I sure miss my beautiful son. I've read and heard people say that losing your child is the worst thing you can ever experience, and I can't disagree. I'd also assumed it would kill me.

At this stage I realize that all these events were horrific but not that unusual, and certainly more are to come. More? All of us will surrender our health, our standing, our marbles, our self soon enough, or so I've been given to understand. Yet the most forceful and eloquent part of my soul still insists I will be the exception. I'm still alive, after all.

Mind you, I do understand the basic biological facts, and I do not believe in the soul. I was raised Roman Catholic, of course, but have spent the last forty years as a secular humanist. Folks like me get branded unbelievers, atheists, heretics, educrats, ethical relativists, Jews, Brights, effete blue-state feminists, eggheaded patched-tweed-and-rimless-bifocals-wearing faggots, French, and much worse; more affectionate terms include freethinker, agnostic, lapsed Catholic, progressive, existentialist, reader of novels, queer, beatnik, and honorary Jew. I'm not sure which label fits best, but I do have a great deal of faith that our bodies—our brainwaves and actions, commerce and science and art, words and children—are pretty much all there is to us. Religion evolved to help us cope with poverty, imprisonment, fear of death, and other bad things, and that's fine. But is some white-bearded guy named Jehovah or Olodumare, God or Allah, really out there? In here? On a throne up in heaven, above and to the left of Cloud 9? Or is he perpetually verging a gazillionth of a nanometer beyond the periphery of a cosmos expanding at 299,792,458 meters per second, frantically tap dancing along the edge of this most naked of all singularities? Was his word, his final solution, on eros, ethics, weaponry, territorial boundaries, contraception, evolution, and somatic cell nuclear transfer inked onto crinkly multilingual papyrus manuscripts a millennium or two ago? My answer to all these is, "Please." I also have faith that there ain't no infernal conflagration after death (unless you want to count the forging of my cremains), no purgatorial scorching of my incorporeal personhood, no seventy-two black-eyed virgins or eighteen choirs of nineteen-year-old lingerie-modeling Brazilo-Scandinavian cherubim waiting on me up in paradise. Nor will I be reincarnated as a wild but eventually Triple Crown–winning black stallion; a granite-jawed southpaw with a 101 mph cutter I can paint the black of the plate with; or the twenty-third century's Abraham Lincoln, let alone its most potent singer-songwriter-guitarist. Even my hero Dante Alighieri's sizzling twelve-year-old girlfriend, Beatrice Portinari, won't *really* be spinning around no Empyrean in perfect equilibrium with Him. (Sorry, D.) Because once my blipping EEG line goes flat, it's going to be all she wrote. In the meantime, my life will be sweet in a number of aspects, a boot in the testicles other times. Sooner or later a Hummer will squash me like Wile E. Coyote. Either that or my heart and maybe another vital organ or two will break down and I'll suffer, piss and moan not a little, then purchase the farm. I've already made the down payment.

As far as the suffering goes—how soon it starts, how long it drags out—I used to be confident that what's called Western medicine was riding full speed, or almost that fast, to the rescue. I knew Western medicine consisted of millions of creative, altruistic, expensively educated women and men, many working in laboratories and hospitals and clinics well to the east and south, but sometimes the term made me picture a single Asian cowgirl in snowy white lab coat and Stetson, bandolier of specimen vials jangling against her modest cleavage as she clutches in one hand the reins of a galloping stallion, in the other a glass pipette delicate enough to boink a healthy cell into the place of a sick one. In another daydream, she wields a titanium lasso delicate enough to snare a 15 mm polyp three and a half feet up my rectum, her motto tattooed in racy arabesque just below either her navel or the base of her spine: *Time to cowgirl up, take your medicine.*

Not that I expected Western medicine to let me live forever— just an extra decade or so, with a little more spring in my step. What I really *really* wanted, daydreams aside, was for people like my daughter Bridget, who has suffered from juvenile diabetes for twenty-two years, to get a fair shot at their biblical threescore and ten. But in August 2001, as Mohamed Atta and Osama bin Laden and Khalid Sheikh Mohammed finalized their plans, our Bible-totin' president, squinting out from his sun-blasted spread down in Crawford, took it upon himself to forbid further use of embryonic stem cells in the effort to cure diabetes, Parkinson's, cancer, MS, and a dozen other vicious diseases. Pretending to split the difference between ultraconservative Christians and the rest of us, the president's "compromise" effectively amounted to a ban on embryonic stem cell research. He said that "more than sixty genetically diverse stem cell lines already exist" and that the NIH would be permitted to fund research on these existing lines only. Less than a dozen of them would ever be made available to scientists, most of them genetically limited to people who tend to use in vitro clinics—the white, the infertile, the wealthy. Not that there's anything innately wrong with these categories, but researchers will need thousands of lines, perhaps even one for every patient, to provide genetic matches for the entire population.

Bush claimed to have given biomedical research "a great deal of thought, prayer, and considerable reflection," but in one fell swoop he'd dammed the flow of a decade of medical research robustly encouraged by President Clinton and a host of Nobel laureates and teaching hospitals. He had stripped my infinitely resourceful cowgirl of her most promising protocol, forcing her to ride sidesaddle on a stubborn Texas mule better equipped to trudge across deserts and oil fields than gallop off into the future. And I couldn't allow that to stand. If this pious, votemongering embarrassment didn't change his position real soon, I might have to do something rash.

In the meantime, in April 2002, a stitch along the left side of my abdomen suddenly graduated into an aching throb. I'd turned fifty-one in late March and was just beginning to get my feet underneath me again after James's death. Life after 9/11 was quite a bit easier to cope with, for me, by comparison. I had tenure as a lit and writing professor, my second marriage was flourishing, and my book about poker was scheduled to be published the following March. While making final revisions to the book and teaching my Literature and Science of Poker class, I felt pretty good about things, as long as you didn't count the abscess in my soul where my son lived.

But within a couple of days the thorn in my side, as I thought of it, had me walking hunched over like a little old man with bad knees and end-stage cirrhosis, not exactly the image I like to project to the world. I much prefer to swagger from success to success like a book-learnt but still macho cowboy: bowlegged, big-cocked, in saddle-worn denim—denim *not* broken in or sandblasted ahead of time by underpaid foreigners. As the throbbing intensified, I gulped down more Advil and prayed—I mean, worried. I'd been taking Zocor, which helped lower my elevated bad cholesterol, for almost two years, this while neglecting to get my liver function tested. Lynn Martin, my primary care physician, had told me to have it checked after three months on the statin because the possible side effects included "nephritis and liver damage," but I somehow forgot. I knew I'd been drinking too much and dosing myself far too liberally with Advil for headaches and hangovers, so my self-diagnosis was "liver failure," though the phrase I used with my wife, Jennifer, was "some liver thing."

Scared by the fatal possibilities but also of hearing them confirmed by Dr. Martin, I finally at Jennifer's insistence made an appointment at our HMO's lab to have my liver enzymes tested. I also stopped drinking—not unheroically, I decided—and, "in spite of the crippling pain," as I phrased it to myself, stopped taking Advil, even though I understood the damage was already done. "Oh, and another thing, Braino," Jennifer said after kissing me, wishing me luck, and dropping me off at the lab. "Your liver's on your right side, not on your left."

Dr. Martin was booked or on vacation, and the first appointment I could get was with her partner Dennis Hughes. Tallish, maybe forty, all business, Hughes glanced at the blood test results, felt around where I'd told him it hurt, asked a few questions, and told me I probably had diverticulitis. "Your liver's functioning perfectly." On the crinkled foot-wide sheet of sanitary paper I'd just been sitting on, he sketched a penisless outline of his patient that featured instead a detailed blowup of my large intestine, complete with hairpin turns and what looked to be wormholes mottling the inner walls. "Diverticulosis. Quite common in people your age." What the hell was that supposed to mean? As I stood there squinting down at my elderly intestines, Hughes continued, "When a seed or food particle gets trapped in one of the holes and becomes infected, it's called diverticulitis." I nodded. *Diiiiiiii-ver-tic-u-liiiiiiiiiiiiiii-tis*, I couldn't help thinking, as the little old woman from Brooklyn used to funnily pronounce it on Letterman. And now here I was, in my unfunny new demographic.

Hughes e-mailed scrips for painkillers and antibiotics to my Walgreens and secured me an appointment for a CT scan of my abdomen, which would confirm his diagnosis. "The colonoscopy two weeks later will confirm that it's all healed up nicely." I nodded. Had I missed something? The practice had just been computerized, and Hughes was happy to demonstrate how my records, medications, new prescriptions, CT appointment, and so on, were "all in the system. The referrals for your scan and colonoscopy are already at Evanston Hospital."

"Terrific."

The antibiotics killed the infection, or at least the symptoms, in a couple of days, so I was able to squirrel the unused painkillers into my party stash. When I called in to report the good news, a nurse reminded me I still needed to get a colonoscopy, just to make sure. "Dr. Martin says you needed to get one anyway."

"I'll make the appointment soon as I hang up," I told her, then sat down to breakfast, all better.

Days went by. Maybe a week. The pain was long gone, and I'd heard all about colonoscopies. You fasted for two or three days while slurping battery acid; step two involved a fully articulated four-foot-long aluminum bullwhip with a searchlight, a video camera, and a lasso at the tip getting launched a few feet up into your large intestine while you watched on a monitor. Not to worry, however. They used really super-duper lubrication.

While discussing some unrelated business with Lewis Lapham, the editor of *Harper's*, I happened to mention my little gastrointestinal adventure. Next thing I knew, Lewis was proposing that I go to the Mayo Clinic for what he called their executive physical, then write a big story about it. Now, this was a guy who had already changed my life for the good and forever by sending me to cover the 2000 World Series of Poker, so I had every reason to trust him—in spite of the fact that he'd aggressively promoted Ralph Nader's run for the presidency in 2000, effectively electing

George Bush. Yet the Mayo proposal triggered a whirlwind of panic about the state of my health. Accepting this plummy assignment would more or less guarantee I'd be told things I did not want to hear. *The good news, Mr. McManus, is you've got almost five weeks to live. The bad news is we started counting over a month ago.* Not really a hypochondriac, I was more a putter-off of nonurgent chores. I changed the oil in my car just before trading it in, and religiously made dental appointments on the thirteenth of Never, to keep me from ever forgetting. And look what had happened to Letterman. During a routine checkup, an angiogram revealed he had a blocked artery and needed an emergency quintuple bypass. This was a fifty-two-year-old guy who ran forty miles a week and looked to have about 1 percent body fat, and that was with TV cameras putting an extra ten pounds on him. What if the Mayo clinicians insisted that I needed to have my rib cage sawed open stat, or discovered a tumor the size of a Titleist wedged inoperably between my pons and my creative left hemisphere? What if, *as they certainly would,* they made me swear off alcohol, tasty food, and my nightly postprandial Parliament Light? Or I had to start running 26.2 miles every morning?

I'd just read somewhere, probably at Jennifer's urging, that you're supposed to get two checkups during your twenties, three in your thirties, four in your forties, every other year of your fifties, and once a year after that—assuming you make it that far. I hadn't had one in seven or eight years, maybe longer. I'd also been nagged by Katie Couric, Lynn Martin, Dennis Hughes, the surgeon general, Jennifer, etc., etc., to get a colonoscopy the minute I turned fifty.

Happy birthday to you.
Happy birthday to you.
May a bullwhip with a camera and a lasso be inserted a couple
*   three feet up into dear Jim-my*
Where he makes num-ber two!

It wasn't that I didn't understand how lucky I was to be offered a free Mayo physical; I just had too many other things on my plate—surf and turf, garlic mashed potatoes, baked ziti, the take-out Mekong Fried Pork from the Phat Phuc Noodle Bar. Next to my plate stood a sweating chrome shaker of Grey Goose martinis, and next to that a dusty bottle of '90 Brunello was breathing. But no! Not only would I have to drink gallons of icky stuff before I got reamed good and proper, they'd make me give up all the good stuff! To say nothing of my terror that the verdict might not be all that rosy.

Bottom line? The bout with diverticulitis had forced my slow hand. I couldn't get medical treatment anymore unless I followed up as I'd promised my doctors I would—my referral was *already in the system*, goddammit—unless I got a colonoscopy as part of the Mayo thing. That way I could get everything checked in seventy-two hours, all under one roof, by the best of the best of the best. It was time to cowboy up, take my medicine. Even so, if I didn't have very young children—my daughters with Jennifer were only three and two—their geezer dad might not have signed up for his physical. But as their mother informed me the moment she got wind of Lewis's offer, "That's that."

LOURDES MN

I know a man who killed another with kindness and too much rich food
... It was clearly accidental manslaughter, not murder, for he had never
seen his victim before then, nor heard of him.

—M.F.K. FISHER, *How to Cook a Wolf*

Time-crunched cooks will cheer for these cute Christmas nibbles from
our Test Kitchen staff. They dipped store-bought Salerno Butter
Cookies into a bright green glaze, then added decorated candies to
form festive wreaths.

—*Taste of Home's Quick Cooking*

The first Western medical school was founded at Salerno in the late Middle Ages, when it finally began to dawn on a small group of doctors that illness had natural rather than divine origins. Heavily influenced by Arabs, Byzantine Greeks, and the largest Jewish community in southern Italy, the school's Latin-speaking scholars established a core curriculum based on more than a hundred texts, including works by Hippocrates, Galen, Isaac Judaeus, and Haly Abbas, as well as a ninth-century Arabic medical handbook. Sick people flocked to Salerno, many of them wounded Crusaders, some of whom recovered in time to gallop back into the fray. Before Salerno, the most advanced centers of medicine were monastic infirmaries, where old tonsured monks instructed young tonsured monks in the arts of bloodletting and leech wrangling, but where the most trusted therapies involved scapulars, benedictions, and holy water. (The miraculous advances of Lourdes, we may recall, didn't become available until 1858.) My own Grandma Grace continued to swear by such hooey for sick children and expectant daughters-in-law as the Beatles were invading America. Billions of people still do.

By the early twelfth century, however, the physician Trota of Salerno, known as *magister mullia sapiens* (wise woman teacher), had compiled a body of medical treatises called the *Trotula*, the first systematic investigation of the facts about conception, pregnancy, embryonic development, and childbirth, and a much needed boon to women lucky enough to be treated by its principles. It thus becomes the ur–Western medicine babe book, preceding by quite a few centuries Madame Curie's papers on radium, Gerty Theresa Radnitz Cori's on biochemistry, Jane Addams's *Twenty Years at Hull-House*, and *Dr. Ruth's Guide to Talking About Herpes*.

Yet most of the Salernitan texts applied to both sexes. According to the nutritional handbook *De flore dietarum*, "Clear wine with an elegant bouquet produces clear blood, comforts the heart, lightens the spirit, banishes sadness and cares, and is suitable for every age and temperament." Perhaps the most widely influential guide was *Regimen sanitatis Salernitanum* (Salernitan Regimen of Health), published in 1260. Its rhymed Latin verses recommended light meals, exercise, enemas, laxatives, and avoiding excessive copulation, the last three of which, at least, Grandma Grace would have heartily approved.

One of the brightest guiding lights of modern Western medicine, William Worrall Mayo, studied science in his native England under John Dalton, who in 1803 had formulated the atomic theory of chemistry. Before Dalton reorganized the periodic table according to the weight of the elements, educated people understood atoms in terms of characteristics observable with the five senses: soap atoms were thought to be slippery balls, acid stung because it was made up of barbed hooks, air consisted of miniature springs, and so on. Dalton and students like Mayo eventually helped us make several huge leaps in our understanding of the chemical nature of health.

After sailing to New York in 1845, Mayo was hired as a pharmacist at Bellevue Hospital, where he dispensed things like castor oil and leeches and was paid so little he had to supplement his income with piecework as a tailor. Four years later he moved his burgeoning family to Lafayette, Indiana, where he undertook Dr. Eliezar Deming's sixteen-week course at the Indiana Medical College. Mayo and his 104 fellow students were forced to share a single microscope. This put them one up, however, on students at Harvard Medical School, which wouldn't provide its first microscope for another twenty years.

Mayo's unique education sparked a lifelong passion for chemical analysis, with what might be found by looking deeper—or just to the west. Traveling by horse and buggy in 1854, he left the malarial climes of Indiana and lit out for the brisker weather of the Minnesota Territory to set up a practice. Known as the Little

Doctor because of his five-feet-four stature, he may have been the only one around who used a microscope to make diagnoses. In much the same spirit, he pioneered ovariotomy—making abdominal incisions into ovaries to determine whether tumors were present—and refined the techniques of what was all too accurately called kitchen surgery.

By 1863, Mayo had been appointed examining surgeon of draftees and volunteers for the Union Army in the southern half of the new state of Minnesota, whose draft board was headquartered in Rochester. He soon moved his family there and set up a practice in which he was eventually joined by his sons Will and Charles. When a tornado struck the town in 1883, destroying most houses and commercial buildings, the Mayos worked with Mother Alfred Moes and her Sisters of St. Francis to provide shelter and medical care for the victims. Rochester had no infirmary, so they turned the only building left standing—a dance hall—into a surgical ward. Making do, they kept injured Minnesotans alive. Once the crisis passed, Mother Alfred raised $60,000 to build a hospital and lassoed Dr. Mayo and his sons into serving as its physicians. Saint Marys, their twenty-seven-bed institution, opened in 1889. As other doctors attached themselves to "the Mayos' clinic," the peculiar idea of a group of specialists caring for a large number of patients began to take shape. Common medical records were established by 1907 to serve the five thousand people who flocked there each year. A network of conveyor belts was designed to move X rays and paperwork more efficiently, in conjunction with one of the world's first telephone paging systems.

Doctors from all over the world began to visit and study, leading in 1915 to the Mayo School of Graduate Education, the first institution devoted to training medical specialists. (The three interlocking shields of its logo represent the mutual dependence of clinicians, researchers, and educators.) Among hundreds of other salutary accomplishments, Mayo clinicians received a Nobel Prize, for the use of cortisone, in 1950. In 1994 they pioneered a study of endothelial dysfunction and chest pain, sparing millions of heart patients terrified ambulance rides and hazardous angiograms. More recently, Mayo scientists developed genetic therapies to repair atherosclerosis and began programming stem cells to generate new, healthy blood vessels.

The Rochester campus now has 1.4 million outpatient visits and 321,900 inpatients a year, all of them under the care of 1,626 physicians and scientists, 1,636 residents and fellows, and a staff of more than 26,000. Eighty percent of the patients come from the upper Midwest, 2 percent from outside the United States. At more than fifteen million square feet, the clinic is almost three times the size of the Mall of America, the Gopher State's less useful mecca. Satellite campuses in Scottsdale, Arizona, and Jacksonville, Florida, bring the total number of inpatients to 503,000 per year. But Mayo's influence emanates much, much more widely. Today, just about anywhere in the world, if you're having blood drawn for chemical analysis (not let to rebalance your humours), awaiting the results of a biopsy, having genetic material examined through an electron microscope, or simply lying on something besides your kitchen table while being treated by a specialist, you are benefiting from the Little Doctor's pathfinding spirit.

A month before my appointment, the clinic mailed me its health questionnaire. Had I recently experienced fever, enlarged glands, abnormal nipple discharge, breast lump, skin rash, skin sores, change in sexual drive or performance, excessive bruising, change of a mole, significant headaches, seizures, slurred speech, excessive thirst, hoarseness, double vision, blurred vision, diminished hearing, dizziness, sinus problems, or none? Did I have a known difficulty with a heart valve? Chest pain? Chest pressure? Rapid heartbeats? Irregular heartbeats? How would I rate my stress level, with 1 the lowest, 5 the maximum? I circled the 4. I considered myself fortunate not to be concerned about HIV, AIDS, or other infectious diseases, but I did feel the need to cut down on my alcohol consumption. As a male, I was asked about my last prostate exam ("1 to 2 years" ago) and whether I'd had a vasectomy (No). Had I experienced erectile dysfunction? The options were No, Yes, or Don't Know. Since I'd probably know if the answer was Yes, and the question didn't specify "ever," I thought it made sense to check No.

In an average week, how many minutes of moderately vigorous or vigorous physical activity did I get? Between 241 and 300 minutes, I checked, referring to time spent riding my bicycle. I was able to eat, dress, use the toilet, keep house, climb stairs, bathe, walk, and transport myself, and to take my own medications. I didn't wear dentures or have special dietary needs. I claimed to eat two servings per day of fruits and/or vegetables. I currently lived in a house with my spouse/family. It was me here completing the form. I had traveled outside the United States or Canada but never received a blood transfusion. I suspected I had narrowed coronary arteries, and that my lungs had been adversely affected by twenty-five years of smoking. I fractured my left wrist twice, when I was fourteen (ice hockey) and fifteen (bicycle). Being in a cast all that time during my growth spurt has made my left wrist and forearm noticeably punier than my right, a condition made worse playing one-handed sports like baseball and tennis. My left meniscus was arthroscopically repaired in 1998, whence the three tiny scars near that knee. My tonsils were removed at age two.

As the form paddled deeper into my family's heart of darkness, I was powerless to circle "adopted." My father's heart problems had killed him at sixty-one, and I've been his physical twin (except for his flaming red hair) all my life. Although my Grandpa Jim died at thirty-five and my brother Kevin at forty-one, my other five siblings are fine. At seventy-five ("the same age as the Oscars," as she always reminds us), our mother is still going strong. Two years ago my total cholesterol was 231 (88 for the bad LDL, only 28 for the good HDL), but after eighteen months on Zocor my total was 162, with the LDL down to 68 and HDL up to 44 (130 and 40 are normal). However far I make it past thirty-five without dying, or forty-six without having a stroke or a heart attack, I believe will be pretty much due to these pale orange pills shaped like shields. Long live the posse who invented them!

It's a cheap, easy flight from O'Hare up to Rochester International, but Jennifer and I decided to make a road trip out of it, the first one we'd take with our daughters. At 350 miles, it seemed long enough for a change of scenery but not too taxing for the girls. We left on a muggy August Saturday morning, stopped in Madison for lunch, and spent the night in Onalaska, on the Wisconsin side of the Mississippi, facing the bluffs. Ten years and one month earlier, Jennifer and I had been issued our marriage license in Unalaska, Alaska (pop. 4,200; by far the biggest town in the Aleutians), before being pronounced man and wife by our ship's captain farther north in the Bering Sea. Now here we were in Onalaska—get it? just *one letter* different—toasting the coincidence with the last glass of wine I'd be drinking for several days. "In case you don't make it, you scaredy-cat," Jennifer "joked" as we clinked.

Seven a.m. Monday morning, I present myself at the Executive Health Program desk on the seventeenth floor of the Mayo Building in downtown Rochester, just across the street from our hotel. The EHP cost $250 more than a regular physical, with the extra fee covering what the brochure calls a streamlined yet comprehensive exam designed to be completed in the shortest possible time. Like all Mayo physicals, it will include preventive screening tests, a comprehensive medical history and examination by an internist, and referrals (if necessary) to subspecialists, as well as health risk and lifestyle assessment for physical fitness. A friendly woman hands me an appointment folder: printed schedule, test instructions, plastic jar for a urine sample. I'm to go when I can, then drop it off at Station S in the subway connecting the hospitals.

My first appointment is for 7:30 at Desk C of the Subway Level, for Venipuncture Specimen Collection. I've been fasting since last night at 7:15, and I've taken no aspirin or iron-containing vitamins for a fortnight. My instruction sheet also has a fifty-point exclamation mark to remind me of my colonoscopy Tuesday morning. No solid food for another twenty-four hours—twenty-seven, actually, since I won't come out of anesthesia till tomorrow afternoon. By then we'll be talking almost two full days, two *empty* days, without eating. Black coffee, tea, Jell-O, or clear chicken broth is okay, but forget about cranberry juice or anything of similar hue. "These liquids show red in the colon and can be confused with blood," warns the sheet.

By 8:04, I am two blocks away in the Gonda Building for an electrocardiogram. I line up outside the long row of cubicles with two dozen well-fed executives in their fifties and sixties, all of us shirtless and hungry as electrodes are stuck to our chests.

Then it's back to the Mayo Building for earwax removal. I tell the otorhinolaryngological nurse, Lisa Thoe, that my hearing has deteriorated in the previous decade or so. I can't always tell what my students in the back of the room are saying, and my wife complains she has to repeat herself half the time. Nurse Thoe has me sit back in what looks like a dentist's chair, complete with overhead klieg light and trayful of gougers and diggers. And then in she goes: *crunch, rasp-rasp, scrape, chisel-chisel* . . .

"No earwax in here, Mr. McAnus."

I patiently correct her, then ask, "Are you sure?"

"Sorry. But nope, none at all, Mr. McManus."

"Okay . . ."

She swings her chair and tray around to check my left ear. Same result. Since the problem isn't hygiene, it might be eardrum degeneration, so I'm sent across the hall for a hearing test. Greg Smith, the tall, blond technician, fits me with headphones that have light wands springing out like antennae. Looking through a window and speaking by intercom, he tells me to press a button when I hear the "isophonemes" he'll shoot at me.

Turns out I have excellent hearing, "above normal" levels for healthy *young* ears. My right ear has 100 percent recognition at 40 dB, my left 95. I have a hearing threshold level of 10 dB at 250 Hertz, and under 5 as the frequency moves into the 4,000–6,000 Hertz range. "My wife says the same thing," Smith confides. "It may have to do with our ability or willingness to concentrate on what's being said." Which Jennifer will be unshocked to hear, whatever Hertz level I can hear at.

For my chest X ray, I wait on a bench with a senator from a northern plains state, a genial guy around my age who prefers not to be identified. He seems to be following me from test site to test site, unless it's the other way around. I'm able to say he looks a lot different in a kneelength powder blue bib than he does in the dark, rumpled suits he favors for TV appearances.

Is the executive program elitist? Depends whom you ask. (I don't ask the senator this, mainly because it's clear his focus today is quite personal.) Those whose hard-earned insurance allows them to come here would tend to say no, I will guess, while the obverse would also be true. America seems not to want socialist flatness, wherein everyone gets mediocre health care at best, but neither will we tolerate too wide a gap between haves and have-nots. Most of us accept that certain members of every culture get cared for more lavishly than others, and that this is not always the worst of all possible worlds. Only czarinas and counts got to flush away "night soil" two hundred years ago, but the steady development of royal technology is why just about everyone now gets to sit on a porcelain throne fitted with copper plumbing and triple-ply Charmin. R&D can take years, even centuries, but eventually the benefits trickle down to the rest of us, though I'm the first to admit that this might not be the most fortunate metaphor. Even Honest Republican Abe used an outhouse for most of his life. It wasn't until 1860, decades before Thomas Crapper brought us the Silent Valveless Water Waste Preventer, that Michael Flannigan invented the Fecal Banishment Apparatus, also known as the

Ablutions Assistant. Lincoln himself gave it a test drive in 1862. "Tarnation!" he declared. "Mr. Flannigan's engine could pull the feathers off a goose at twenty paces. For a man standing to relieve himself from a fair distance, this contraption makes it darned near impossible to miss! The lady folk will be most appreciative of that." The president, however, soon had what he believed to be a clairvoyant nightmare in which the device swallowed his son Tad, and he decided against installing one in the White House. Tad's eleven-year-old brother Willie had just succumbed in February to typhoid fever, almost certainly caused by pollution of the capital's water system; many historians also believe that General George McClelland's near-fatal bout with the disease almost sank the Union's cause. So even at the top of our social pyramid, people died of such things in those days.

A couple of summers ago Garrison Keillor, a registered NPR type, found the Mayo to be quite democratic. While it's famous as the clinic where, as he put it, "the Exalted Nawab of Lower Rawalpindi's 14th and 15th wives go in for a chest X ray," Keillor noted that it also quietly serves most of southern Minnesota. His only complaint was that during his checkup he had to wait a lot, and he recommended bringing a book—Dante or the Book of Job. But he called this the Lourdes of the North. For an extra $250, the price of a half-decent Weber grill or a World Series of Poker super-satellite, senators and corporate VPs and *Harper's* reporters don't have to wait quite as long.

"Turn to the right and cough."

I comply. Nothing like knobby male fingers probing your scrotum to mitigate guilt about privileged white maleness. No, sir.

"Okay, that's good."

The doctor in charge of my overall checkup is Donald D. Hensrud. From the earliest days, each Mayo patient has been assigned a personal physician who coordinates access to all clinic services and follow-up treatments. Hensrud's job is to initiate my chart, check my vitals, take a comprehensive history and physical exam, decide whether further tests are appropriate, then integrate the results into an overall prognosis and treatment plan. He has no vested interest in testing for every last thing, or in skipping the pricey tests, either. In this he is following "the spirit of the clinic" established by William J. Mayo in 1921: "Group medicine is not a financial arrangement except for minor details, but a scientific cooperation for the welfare of the sick." All Mayo doctors receive a salary unrelated to the number of exams and surgeries they perform or lab tests they order, and the clinic proudly continues as a not-for-profit, charitable public trust.

"Please kneel down there and lean forward."

Oh boy. Hensrud has almost freakishly wide blue eyes, pale skin, and silver hair parted in the middle, combed back. Midnight blue suit, crisp white shirt, glinting yet sober blue tie. For an extra dash of color, he's wearing a mauve rubber glove, with which he points to a pull-out ledge near the bottom of the examining table. Kneeling down with my back to him feels extra peculiar, perhaps, because he's wearing that suit instead of a lab coat, especially as I tender myself to his application of a cool smear of lubricant. Ew. A moment ago we were having a civilized man-to-man talk, two fully clothed guys with young children, bicycles, wine, and our writing in common. Now Dr. Hensrud has a long, knobby index finger *way* up my rectum, feeling around to gauge, he informs me, the distendedness of my prostate. Finally, *finally,* maybe twelve seconds later, it's over. "Absolutely normal," pronounces my violator as he peels off his maculate glove. "No nodules or enlargement."

"Great," I say, assiduously avoiding eye contact. "Yeah, great."

As I lie faceup on the table, he determines that my venous pressure and jugular reflexes are normal, my carotids without bruits, my lungs clear, my flesh free of edema, and that pulses are palpable in my distant extremities.

Once I've pulled up my boxers, Hensrud directs me to the changing room in the corner. *Yahoo!* Back in my clothes, I emerge a new man through the curtain, ready to resume our conversation as though no orifices had been penetrated.

The fact is, Hensrud's modesty and gravitas make him seem almost saintly—Alyosha Karamazov in pinstripes, with a wallful of high-powered medical diplomas instead of a monastic faith in Orthodox Russky miracles. Two M.S.'s in public health, medical degrees from four universities. He also serves as the medical editor in chief and lead writer of *Mayo Clinic on Healthy Weight*, a book I've been reading all summer.

Referring to the history I mailed in, he pointedly asks whether I've had family or work problems related to alcohol.

"You mean like tavern brawls, wilding . . ."

Patient smile for the defensive patient. "DUI arrests and the like."

"No DUIs, no."

"That's good. How much do you drink?"

On the questionnaire next to "Substances Review: Alcohol; Current use," I recall checking "3–7 days per week," heartened by the Mayo's refusal to make petty distinctions between imbibing every night and every so often. Next to "Previous use," I also checked 3–7 days per week. "Current number of servings per day" provided three options: 1–2, 3–4, and 5–10+. I circled the first two and put my check mark between them, and checked 3–4 next to "Previous use," though I *have* had my fair share of 5–10+ evenings. I also admitted to "using" caffeine 3–7 days per week, 3–4 servings per day. "Current use of tobacco" provided no box for "one daily," so I wrote that in, too; next to "Previous use," I checked "½ to 1 pack per day," and "16–30" as the number of years.

Even while grilling me, Hensrud's tone remains formal but warm, with a throw-his-head-back-to-laugh sense of humor. He makes direct, friendly eye contact, hears out my answers, and speaks in complete sentences and paragraphs. Not that I always want to listen. "When you have family members who develop heart disease this young, especially with your grandfather at thirty-five, we're of course more concerned about it. The fact that your father was a smoker and had type 2 diabetes certainly increased his risk. When I see a family history like this, I ask about other things we maybe haven't checked yet. Homocysteine, for one, a protein in the blood that acts like cholesterol—the higher the homocysteine, the greater the risk of heart disease. Lipoprotein (a)—kind of like cholesterol, in that it increases your risk. Another one is C-reactive protein. We're going to check these to see if they might be elevated."

Thinking of Letterman's bypass, I ask, "Isn't there some machine that can gauge, you know, blood flow?"

"Right now there isn't a noninvasive way to check for narrowing of the arteries. But we're not going to order angiograms on anyone without symptoms, much less somebody who's young and healthy."

I wanted to hug him but managed to restrain myself, in no small part due to the freshness of our proctologic encounter. "What about someone like me, though, who's got the family history, ain't so young anymore, and sometimes feels twinges?"

"Well, first we characterize the chest pain, then we do diagnostic studies. And we emphasize prevention and controlling risk factors, because that's the bottom line anyway. You're not having symptoms, so you aren't a candidate for surgery based on what we think the anatomy might show. Otherwise I would order an angiogram." He picks up a life-size heart model, which I find hard to look at—like it might cause a myocardial infarction psychosomatically. "We'd inject dye into these three arteries to see how much blockage there was. That's the gold standard, though it's highly invasive. And without any symptoms at all, we just don't do angiograms. They're a pretty big deal, which is why they're performed in a hospital. The benefits don't outweigh the risks. You do enough of them, you're going to cause problems in somebody where none had existed before." He puts down the heart. "What we'll do is a coronary calcification study, an ultrafast spiral CT scan of the heart, that looks for calcification in these arteries." He points to the center of his chest, two-thirds of the way up the blue tie. "As plaque builds up and narrows the artery, it calcifies." He knows I got scanned at the University of Illinois five years ago, and he picks up their printout, which I mailed in with the questionnaire. "This is good. You were at the fortieth percentile. Fiftieth percentile would be average, of course, but for heart disease, you don't want to be average, because one of three people will die of it."

"Roger."

I've read in *The Mayo Clinic Heart Book* that cardiovascular disease is the country's number one killer. Not cancer? Not guns or DUIs? Nope, and it's not even close. Heart problems kill more of us than the next *seven* leading causes *combined*. Sixty million Americans are on track to go out in this manner.

"What's good," Hensrud says, "is despite your risk factors, high cholesterol, and family history, you were better than average on this, but you have to remember this test looks at calcification indirectly. What we don't know is whether the plaque has built up in a critical area, or whether it's likely to rupture. It's an imperfect test, though it does give us good information, and in your case it gives us a baseline. We'll give you another one now, compare it with five years ago, and see if there's been major progression."

Next subject: diet. Shamelessly deploying flattery as a goad, Hensrud tells me, "You're already on the right track." Pregnant, professional pause. "I would cut down on your portion size. I hate to say this, but you should also cut back on the pasta, increase the vegetables and fruits . . ."

As he outlines a diet for me, I interrupt to ask what *he* eats.

"I don't want to preach, but if a person asks me, I'll tell him. My lunch every day, I try to get in a lot of fruit. In the evening a salad can become the main part of our meal." He responds to my long face by adding: "People underestimate the ability to change—to like new foods. Think back to the way you ate twenty years ago. You've already cut down on meat, and this is just an extension of that. Eating healthy and eating well are not mutually exclusive. The less animal product you consume the better, but you can still eat a very tasty diet." Italicizing all this is the lean, healthy fitness so evident under the suit, while the suit itself (Prada?) adds to his wiry authority. It probably wouldn't do, after all, to have the Mayo's healthy-weight expert lumbering chubbily through the corridors—Chris Farley in a ketchup-stained lab coat promoting cardiovascular fitness.

There are excellent physicians in every large city—certainly Chicago has an embarrassment of medical riches—but places like Mayo have strength in numbers and the efficiency of a well-integrated system. Hensrud has dozens of world-class experts just down the block, or the hall, to ask or answer questions, so it's easier for everyone to stay up on the literature. Major-league medical conferences take place every day, right on campus.

It's a privilege, of course, to be examined by a doctor who's a leader in his field: who has research ongoing, who publishes his findings in forums like *Cardiology Today and Tomorrow* and *The American Journal of Cardiology*. Even two-year-old research can be much less useful these days, when the state of the art is advancing so rapidly. It matters less to me that Hensrud consults for ABC News, *Fortune* magazine, and Blue Shield of California than that he literally wrote the book about how a person with my cardiovascular issues should eat and take care of himself. Like most people, I don't require the steadiest (and priciest) surgical hand guiding a laser through my ventricles—yet. I need to be told by someone I respect what to eat and drink and what not to, and which medications to take. Not that a lesser doc would scan my test results and put me on a diet of deep-fried chimichangas and blue agave tequila, but when a Mayo clinician is doing the nudging, the message may finally get through.

"Okay. Now I need your permission to drink a little wine of an evening."

"Okay," he says warily, "but let me ask you a question."

Uh-oh. "Shoot."

"Do you think you're self-medicating, or you've ever done that in the past?"

While I blush, hem, and stutter, he draws me a lazy, rounded-off J with no crossbar, calling it the J-shaped curve. "The vertical axis represents overall mortality, the horizontal is alcohol consumption. Moving left to right, people who consume moderate amounts have a lower risk of dying early than people who don't consume any at all. But once you start drinking a lot, mortality steeply ascends."

"What do you mean by 'a lot'?"

"That's the million-dollar question. Risk of dying increases because of other stuff you do when you're drinking too much. Cardiovascular disease stays pretty flat, but the risks of liver cancer, homicide, and accidents all go way up."

I tell him I've heard *moderate* defined as one to two drinks a day, a drink being six ounces of wine, twelve ounces of beer, or one ounce of hard stuff.

"On average, Jim. On average."

"You're saying I can have seven to fourteen glasses of wine a week?!"

A brief, slightly exasperated pause, before: "Yes."

Hallelujah! "Okay then," I tell him.

"Even so, I'm a little nervous when you talk about 'every day' because people get into a habit and habits can sneak up and bite you." By *bite*, he means torture you with cirrhosis and stroke and then kill you. By *people*, he means the perfect J-shaped curve slumped in front of him. "I'd also recommend going for a period of time without alcohol, as a reality check. Whether that's once or twice a week or periodically throughout the year—if it's a problem going without it that long, then it's a problem by definition."

Finally, he pulls up my blood studies on his big, flat PC screen. They drew the blood less than three hours ago, but W. W. Mayo's focus on chemistry and intra-clinic communication are still much in evidence. And Hensrud is happy to tell me my hemoglobin level is "fine." No problems, either, with anemia or blood count. White cells, platelets, iron levels, thyroid, and urine—all fine. Normal electrocardiogram. After a quarter century of smoking and a decade popping beta carotene, my chest X ray revealed only slight fibrosis in my lower lungs, which is "nothing to worry about." Exhale. "Your PSA, the prostate blood test, is perfect: 1.1. Normal is up to 2.9. Slightly elevated levels of uric acid, 8.9. Normal is 4.3 to 8." My AST liver test is 34. Normal is 12 to 31, but Hensrud isn't concerned. "Tiny elevation, that's all." My blood sugar is 90—normal is 70 to 100—so there's no evidence yet of impending diabetes.

"Total cholesterol is 165," he continues. "Average for men in this country is 205. That you're forty points below is probably due to the Zocor. But your triglycerides are still at 462, so you've got what we call dyslipidemia. The HDL [high-density lipoprotein] cholesterol is 34, a little too low. When the triglycerides are this high, we can't even calculate the bad LDL. Triglycerides are volatile; they bounce around more. I'd be absolutely more concerned about cholesterol of 462 than triglycerides of 462. You haven't developed high blood pressure or an elevated glucose count, which is great, but I think you have a slightly greater risk of developing them because of your family history. It's the classic pattern: alcohol, sugar, and weight. Just remember, whatever efforts you put in from now on will be directly proportional to the results you see. My sense is that it would be counterproductive for me to tell you to stop drinking wine and eating sweets. That's ridiculous. Make whatever changes you can live with comfortably, then we'll start working on the medication side of things."

I tell him I've been watching my caloric intake for years, exercising almost every day. "I could certainly drink a lot less, and I plan to, but I'd also like to be somewhat more aggressive with medication."

This last doesn't please Alyosha. "My best recommendation would be to make whatever changes you can on your own before we change medication. Because the risk of side effects would go way up, I'm a little more hesitant to use combination therapy."

"What about boosting the Zocor?"

"That's a possible option. At higher doses, Zocor tends to lower triglycerides a little bit and raise HDL a little bit more. But again, you'd be increasing the chances of side effects. The overall risk of liver problems is less than one half of 1 percent, but it increases with dose. All of the statins—except maybe Pravachol—can cause myositis or muscle breakdown that can be fatal, though it's very uncommon. Again, I'm not asking you to do anything heroic. I'm just saying, let's see how much we can get from comfortable lifestyle changes, then see where we're at."

It's a plan.

Because of my age, positions of influence, birth order (first of seven), and other factors, I tend to trust those in authority. Whether I'm buying a car or a puppy, a novel or a computer, I'm content to deliver myself into the hands of an expert. Instead of spending decades learning Russian with run-of-the-mill comprehension, I count on Richard Pevear and Larissa Volokhonsky for versions of *Anna Karenina* and *The Brothers Karamazov* more subtle and poetic than I could ever in a hundred years hope to come up with on my own. The time I save not trying to parse Count Lev's upper-caste syntax or Fyodor Mikhailovich's born-again slavophile ravings, to say nothing of the Cyrillic alphabet, allows me to also read *The Mahabharata*, *The Iliad*, *My Name Is Red*, and *Love in the Time of Cholera*, albeit in translation. Not that the world wouldn't be a better place if I mastered Sanskrit, Homeric Greek, modern Trojan, and Colombian Spanish and thus partook of those cultures directly; on the other hand, bro, life is short. (If it wasn't, why invite digits and digital video cameras to be launched up your rectum?) It's for much the same reason I don't cram for the MCAT, attend and pay for medical school, then do a six-year gastroenterology residency when I come down with diverticulitis: because any board-certified specialist worth her sodium chloride knows infinitely better than I ever could what sort of shape my intestines are in, better still how to heal them.

One obvious downside of this way of thinking is that millions of postmenopausal women who took estrogen with progestin were following the same logic, and they were often fatally misled. We didn't find this out until the summer of 2002, after the Department of Health underwrote the Women's Health Initiative's randomized control trial, which showed that the numbers who developed breast cancer, heart attacks, strokes, or blood clots in the lungs were *higher* on the E plus P regimen.

Likewise, the Cardiac Arrhythmia Suppression Trial reexamined the conventional wisdom that certain antiarrhythmia drugs helped prevent second heart attacks. The trial involved 1,500 heart attack victims: half received antiarrhythmics while the other 750 were slipped a placebo. These mortally vulnerable patients thus had the same odds of getting the lifesaving therapy as they'd get on the pass line of a craps table. How darned unfortunate, then, to be randomly shunted into the placebo group, condemned to crap out by a computerized roll of the dice! Yet researchers have to break eggs to make omelets, right? And so, in the interest of medical science, the trial was scheduled to run for at least two years. The early results were so dramatic, however, that it was halted after only ten months for the health of the unlucky guinea pigs. Those patients knocking back a sugar pill each morning, in the innocence of their already damaged hearts, were found to be about two and a half times more likely to *survive* than those taking the antiarrhythmic.

I've personally downed thousands of little gold vitamin E capsules for the good of my arteries. Who sanctioned this regimen? I can't say exactly, but I think of it as having "floated" to me through "the culture." In any case, I was misled. And then, having smoked cigarettes for a quarter of a century, I snatched at another flotation device by dosing myself with the antioxidant beta carotene to decrease my risk of lung cancer. Now I'm told by experts that beta carotene *increases* my chances of developing that form of cancer.

Two generations ago, doctors smoked cigarettes in TV commercials, and people with my genes and habits bought the farm even younger. It also turns out that if you were born in the northern hemisphere during the month of May, you're 13 percent more likely to develop multiple sclerosis. Better to be born in November, according to Professor George Ebers of the Radcliffe Infirmary at Oxford University. In other words, if you have a family history of MS, it's best to make procreative love during February. On Valentine's Day, for example, after exchanging cards dappled with pink hearts and cutely drawn demyelinated nerve fibers. But when should a heart patient do it?

As the lovesick postman in *Il Postino* shrugs pathetically, "I was confused."

In the meantime, though, here I am navigating postmodern Lourdes. As the Mayos and their architects anticipated, no healthy person, let alone someone who's mortally ill, wants to traipse through a Minnesota winter from appointment to appointment, so they put in a subway system and fitted it with chandeliers, Chihuly flowers, and enormous glass panels near the top, facing south to let in extra sunshine, while in August the mega AC compressors make everything pleasanter. What a great day, I decide, to be . . . eating.

The refrigerator back up in the twelfth-floor executive lounge is stocked with complimentary mineral water, fruit juice, and instant bouillon and chicken broth. Dizzy, I tear open a foil packet of pee-yellow slime and let it drip down into a styrofoam cup of hot water, watching it curl up like smoke from a cyanide popper. *Buon appetito!*

In my room at the Kahler Grand Hotel Monday evening, I knock back my first dose of Fleet Phospho-Soda, a putatively ginger-lemon-flavored oral saline laxative. That is, I try to. After mixing 1.5 ounces into a half-full glass of water, I take my first sip. If the Dead Sea's a 2 on the icky continuum, and King Oscar sardine juice a 3½, Fleet Phospho-Soda is at the very, very least an 11.

The trick is to get as much of it down my throat while tasting as little as possible, mainly by pouring it past the more sensitive taste buds near the front of my palate. I plop in four ice cubes and click on the television, settling back with my cocktail of little barbed hooks. So as not to tempt dear old dad, Jennifer and the girls are dining downstairs in the restaurant; our suite also provides separate bedrooms, an excellent thing for reasons I'll address in a minute. The girls had a wonderful day exploring Rochester and environs, especially the old-time movie theater converted into a Barnes & Noble with a vast children's section. The only downside, according to Jennifer, was the heartbreaking horror show of terminally ill children being wheeled back and forth between hospitals. She had a lot of hard questions to answer.

One place they probably won't want to visit tomorrow is the Rochester Federal Prison, a "country-club facility" (according to my complimentary issue of *Rochester Magazine*) just up the road that until recently housed longtime Chicago congressman Dan Rostenkowski. Other guests have included perennial candidate Lyndon LaRouche, nutjob evangelist Jim Bakker, broomstick-wielding rapist Justin Volpe, the only FBI agent ever convicted of first-degree manslaughter (Mark Putnam, for strangling an informant), and Clyde Bellecourt, who occupied the Bureau of Indian Affairs in Wounded Knee, South Dakota. Currently on hand in the facility is Sheik Omar Abdel Rahman, the blind colleague of Osama bin Laden who sanctioned the Islamists who gunned down Anwar Sadat, detonated bombs outside our embassies in Africa, targeted landmarks and humans all over New York and Cairo, and managed to strike the World Trade Center in 1993 and 2001. Many of these attacks must have been spiritually encouraged from his comfy cell right here in Rochester.

Mayo doctors and their unholy Western medicine continue to help Abdel Rahman avoid further deterioration of his eyes and internal organs, though it cannot be easy for them. It has been reported that one doctor placed a hand gently on his shoulder, her usual way of establishing rapport with blind patients. When the sheik wrathfully brushed her off, she apologized, adding that she'd meant it only as a gesture of friendship and respect. "If you respected me," Abdel Rahman said, "you would know that a woman in my culture would never dare touch a man!" Wincing and sipping my Fleet, I try to imagine the human touch a violently rabble-rousing Christian or Jewish cleric would receive in a Muslim penitentiary.

If their numbers along Mayo corridors and on sidewalks downtown are any indication, Arabs and Muslims are certainly made to feel welcome in Rochester. This hotel has a five-page menu of Middle Eastern cuisine printed in Arabic. Hanging with the Stars and Stripes in the dome above the rooftop pool are the flags of Saudi Arabia, Jordan, Oman, United Arab Emirates, and Turkey, along with those of Mexico, Australia, and the Seychelles. The cable TV package includes four Arabic stations. Right now Channel 63 is showing a huge crowd swirling around a black glyph in what must be Mecca, with close-ups of worshipers chanting their prayers; the station's logo on the screen's upper left is a palm tree emerging from a pair of crossed scimitars. Al Jazeera is on Channel 64. Next time I click there, enraged Palestinians are bearing a bloodied young man on a stretcher.

Watching this helps pass the time between limping sprints to the bathroom. By 8:37, I'm down to short blasts of ginger-lemon fizz and shorter, more parched emanations—or as Dante wrote of another inferno, *ed elli avea del cul fatto trombetta* ("and he made a trumpet of his ass"). Meanwhile, Arabest News on Channel 65 has mountainous battlefield footage from what must be Kashmir. Channel 66 has a soap opera: men without beards, women in chic clothes and hairstyles. An anchor in a Western business suit reads the news on Al Jazeera next to footage of Vladimir Putin.

Our own president, as it happens, underwent a colonoscopy by a Navy GI at Camp David a few weeks before mine. Two benign polyps had been discovered while he was governor of Texas, and this last procedure was part of the standard follow-up. Given a choice of local anesthesia and mild sedation or a general anesthesia with Propofol, Mr. Bush chose the latter regime. Before going under at 7 a.m., he invoked the 25th Amendment, transferring power to Vice President Dick Cheney just in case, for example, Saddam or Osama took the opportunity to lob a few Scuds at the Halliburton derricks in the exurbs of Riyadh or Fort Worth while the " ' "*real*" ' " commander in chief was sedated. The only previous invocation of this amendment came in 1985, when Ronald Reagan had surgery for colon cancer and George H. W. Bush *not Alexander Haig, damn it* was in charge for seven hours and fifty-four minutes, paving the way for Bush 41 to become, in a sense, a two-term president himself. It remains to be seen whether the same colorectal pretext will work for Mr. Cheney.

Naval colonoscope was withdrawn from presidential sphincter at 7:29, and Mr. Bush came to at 7:31. Most doctors check their patient's post-anesthesia alertness by asking who the president of the United States is, but though we're told Mr. Bush's GI, Air Force colonel Richard Tubb, chose an equally obvious question, we haven't been told what it was. Perhaps he asked, "What's

the capital of Grecia?" or "Wasn't Cruise awesome in *Top Gun?*"
In any event, by 9:24, after tossing a ball for his dogs and scarfing
a plate of waffles, the president was back, so to speak, in the saddle, ready to bushwhack any godless stem cell research, sign a
more fair and balanced tax code, and then—saving the best for
the last—decide who gets to be the ace of spades on his cool
desert-camouflage poker deck.

IMPEDANCE
PLETHYSMOGRAPHY

Your heart is a muscular pump the size of your fist. Located to the left of the center of your chest, its lower tip points to the left.

—*Mayo Clinic Heart Book*

Are you paying attention to my heartbeat? A real doctor's or nurse's stethoscope. Pliable nylon tubing and shiny stainless steel ear piece. A great toy and finishing touch to any uniform.

—www.erosboutique.org

Tuesday morning at 4:45 my wake-up call announces it's time for my second round of Fleet, just in case any 2 mm shreds of Onalaska walleye managed to withstand the forced evacuation last night. This time I cheat by diluting the stuff with twice the recommended volume of water, but it still ain't the perkiest beverage to help you greet Dawn's rosy fingers, let alone your gastroenterologist's. Must be why this is called the asshole-to-breakfast-time checkup.

After ninety minutes of CNN, Fleet, Al Jazeera, no breakfast, and a shower interrupted by my umpteenth scalding sit-down, I hustle four blocks to the Eisenberg Building, check in, and dash to the men's room. Reemerging eight minutes later, I submit to yet another blood pressure cuff and digital ear thermometer, declining advice about a living will before dashing to the men's room. Soon I am ushered into a deeper, more sterile waiting area, which has its own men's room, thank God.

My only fellow waiter this morning is a large, chatty black man from Kansas City. As naturally as if we're placing the Royals and White Sox on the abysmal continuum, we start shooting the . . . breeze about colon health, HMOs, Fleet preps. The young man—he tells me he's thirty-six—shakes his head in wonder to hear that I had to down only one glassful of Phospho-Soda per session, for a total of two, then makes me repeat myself to see if he heard right the first time. For some reason, his prep required one glassful *every fifteen minutes for three and a half hours*. Worse, this is his "ninth or tenth" colonoscopy. His father and two of his uncles died early, and he himself has already had "dozens" of polyps removed. He does not use the C word but says that depending on what they discover this morning, the Mayo GI team will probably advocate removing his entire colon, which will mean "wearing the bag" for the rest of his life. A string of clichés about "these days" and "all their advances" is the best I can manage to encourage him. When they call his name first, we shake hands, don't smile, and wish each other good luck.

Ten minutes later Lawrence Szarka is looming above me in the chrome-and-glass dazzle of endoscopy Suite No. 2, because what other room would they put me in? We're surrounded by EKG and video monitors, a pneumatic tube portal for biopsy specimens, and right here, up close, atop Szarka's instrument table, a colonoscope coiled like a silvery Mapplethorpe bullwhip. Am I ready for this? We will see. I lie on my side, semi-fetal, with my back to the doc, watch the nurse pump 100 mcg fentanyl and 5 mg midozolam into the back of my hand, and wake up thirsty in the recovery room.

Wha happeh?

What happened was that soon after I passed out at 8:10, a second nurse, Marcia Ward, applied a liberal dose of Novaplus lubricant to patient McManus's anus, through which Dr. Szarka inserted the Olympus PCF-160AL variable-stiffness pediatric colonoscope. For the last two years, he and his fellow GIs at Mayo have been using kiddy colonoscopes on most mature patients. The PCF-160 is leaner, more flexible than the standard adult model, but in the right hands it still gets the job done. Guided by the camera and lamp at its tip, Szarka advanced the scope into my cecum, which he identified on the monitor in front of him by the presence of the appendiceal orifice and the ileocecal valve. Clean and clean. He intubated my terminal ileum (also known as the Sac of Troy) for a distance of 5 cm and observed it was normal. The mucosa in my sigmoid colon (named, of course, for the Viennese punk power trio founded and disbanded by the radical grammarian Hans X) had scattered small diverticula, also normal for a person my age. Szarka also observed that my bowel preparation was excellent, thank you very much, and that so far I was tolerating the procedure quite manfully. If I could have, we would have touched fists.

The *aha* moment came after Szarka had reached an anatomically difficult hairpin turn in my sigmoid colon, in which he spotted some protuberant tissue. No, not my head. Just a polyp. Assisted by Ward, he passed an electrocautery snare through the scope, positioned it above the polyp, and lowered the lasso loop over it. Ward pulled the snare's other end until she and Szarka could see on the monitor that the lasso had tightened around the base of the polyp. By pressing a foot pedal that sent twenty joules of energy through the snare, Szarka cauterized the base of the polyp while pulling the rest of it away from the wall of my colon. When he told Ward to cut, she tugged on the trigger device, which snipped off the polyp by closing the snare all the way. Szarka then suctioned the damn thing back out through the channel and into the light. Fifteen millimeters long, it was about the size and consistency of a shiitake stem pickled in sake. He dropped it into a specimen container, which Ward slid into the tube portal behind her, from which point it was sucked over to the Department of Laboratory Medicine and Pathology in the Hilton Building, three blocks away. Data gathered during these procedures are transmitted electronically, of course, but you still need a three-dimensional tube to convey biological specimens. Mayo's pneumatic pipeline was installed in the 1930s to more efficiently relay files and lab samples around the campus; these days the system is controlled on a Windows NT platform. Over in Pathology, a technician sectioned the polyp and applied a stain of hematoxylin-eosin; without the stain, such tissue cannot be visually distinguished from an adenomatous polyp, the sort that can become cancerous. Following once again in the footsteps of W. W. Mayo, pathologist Susan Abraham would soon slide the specimen under a microscope and make her diagnosis. In the meantime, back in Suite No. 2, Dr. Szarka found the rest of my colon, including a retroflexed view of my rectum, to be normal, though the PCF-160 provided only circumscribed views as to whether or not I was anal.

Once the IV was removed from my hand at 8:36, an orderly wheeled me down the hall to recovery, where I came to a little before 9. No, I could not have some water. I'd been warned in advance that my memory might get a bit dicey; it did. I may have fallen asleep again, too, but at some point a glance at my schedule reminds me I need to have blood drawn again before eating. Released from recovery at 10:26, I resume my executive powers.

With my appetite all the way back, I hustle over to Station C for my second venicultural shanking. Even dizzier now, I dash to the main cafeteria. Noshing greedily the first of two turkey sandwiches washed down with cranapple juice, I review the post-exam symptoms I've been advised to watch out for. These include bleeding from the rectum, a temperature above 100.4, and persistent rectal or abdominal pain "that is not relieved by expelling gas." In an effort to sense bloody moisture, I clench my buttocks while rocking side to side on the chair, since reaching behind me to put my fingers down there in the middle of a brightly lit cafeteria would not speak well of me. No. Pressing the back of my hand to my forehead seems acceptable, though, as does a septet of hushed, modest farts. In each respect, I seem to be fine.

In the Division of Allergy and Outpatient Infectious Disease, a tall dirty-blond Minnesota R.N. immunizes me against typhus and diphtheria, and advises me to get flu shots each autumn and to "keep track of Hep A and Hep B." Instead of inquiring how one goes about this, I nod, take a bite of my sandwich.

Next stop, a one o'clock consult with Peggy A. Menzel, R.D. My continually updated e-chart refers to me now as "an executive male referred for medical nutrition therapy, weight control, and hypertriglyceridemia," nine speedy syllables for *way* too much fat in my bloodstream. Scarcely 68 inches tall, I weigh in at a whopping 85.28 kilograms, or 188.01 pounds.

"If only I could lose that last hundredth . . ."

"Alcohol," quizzes Menzel, "with a typical dinner?"

"Oh, a couple-three glasses of wine, I would say. If we go to a restaurant, we sometimes start off with martinis . . ."

Wrong answer.

" 'Martinis . . .' Dessert?"

Yet another wrong answer.

Menzel's advice contains few surprises, though it must be a good thing that everyone at Mayo is on the same page. I should eat more fruits and vegetables, fewer carbohydrates and sweets, drink much more water and much *much* less alcohol. My single serving of meat or fish "should never be larger than a deck of cards," proportions with which I'm familiar. If I want something sweet with or after dinner, I should have some fresh fruit. Grey Goose L'Orange and Stoli Limon are no longer suitable substitutes.

By 1:45, I'm a couple of underground blocks away in the Baldwin Building, Division of Cardiovascular Diseases, for my treadmill test. The sandwiches and juice have me feeling a lot more like myself. Jessica Schliep, the athletic blond cardiopulmonary technician and Certified Exercise Specialist assigned to my case, whispers, "Take off your shirt for me, please." She doesn't really whisper, of course.

Wishing I'd done 700,000 more push-ups and crunches last night, I comply. But maybe these young CES's *like* chubby hubbies, and not just because we're keeping them in business. Because what about Biggie Smalls, Tone Loc, the guy in Blues

Traveler, and Tony Soprano? According to the deconstruction-istas, *The Sopranos* is a "feminist metatext," male fatness "a signi-fier with many overlapping and even contradictory signifieds . . ."

On the subject of significant overlap, Jessica wrenches and twists my left love handle in her surprisingly strong right hand, flexing a jumbo caliper in her left to gauge the diameter. Think *that* was humiliating? A contrary feminist's meta-assault on my middle-aged straight white male manhood? Because now she is brandishing a three-bladed cartridge, looking my torso up and down while picking her spots, and not particularly liking what she sees, I'm afraid. After shaving a few hairs, she uses an emery board to sand down a thumbnail-size patch of skin on my chest. Then she does it again, and again, and *again*, for a total of fifteen little patches running diagonally from my sternum across my left ribs to a pair up near my left armpit, another on my back, and another on my neck. And each and every last time it *oits!*

With the heartbreakingly freckled bridge of her nose an inch from my chin, she proceeds to stick an electrode on each smart-ing spot, expertly plugging the opposite ends of the insulated wires into a black distributor attached to the belt she's now busy securing around my waist, all this as a loony temptation arises to reach up and, at the very, very least, pat her shoulder. Good job! So thank God a second, more highly credentialed technician chooses this moment to walk in and take charge of the scene. She, too, is lithe and attractive, right down to her slim-cut black tracksuit and racy, albeit low-heeled, Nike cross-trainers. Jodie L. Lester, CES, says her badge.

"Hello, Mr. McManus."

"Hello, Jodie. And please call me Jim."

Not one for small talk either, Jodie tells Jessica to prepare the

Bruce protocol, then crisply orders me onto on a pricey-looking exercise contraption. "Keep your feet apart, straddling the tread-mill, then step down onto it as soon as I push the start button."

Dungeons in Paris and Amsterdam, I've heard, as well as in other Sodoms and Gomorrahs of Olde Europe, charge upwards of six hundred euros for a two-mistress session. Thousands more stipulate on the Internet to being outfitted with nurse uniforms, violet wands, tourniquets, speculums, Wartenberg pinwheels, Jennings oral retractors, and other paraphernalia conducive to "medical and electroplay scenarios with happy outcomes." Even as a proud blue-state resident, I confess to being morally outraged by such perverse and concupiscent advertising, and plan to write my congressman stat; I may even put my money where my mouth is by canceling our blazingly fast broadband service, or trading down somewhat from my thirty-seven-inch Active Matrix TFT with four-mode VESA DPMC monitor. Yet there's no way these virtual dungeons could offer more striking personnel and scenarios than the Mayo does right here in Rochester, especially if your woefully vanilla stress test should prove inconclusive the first time. In this case your doctor might order a strain-gauge plethys-mography, for example, during which the cruel CES wraps a blood pressure cuff around your leg, extra tight. Or why not sub-mit to transcutaneous oximetry, particularly if you cotton to the idea of electrodes being taped to your sandpapered skin, the bet-ter for Jessica to appraise your oxygen diffusion? Your HMO or magazine editor may even spring for a Doppler ultrasound, in which the "doctor" listens to the whoosh of your blood through a transducer, whose erotic utility I can only begin to imagine. Per-haps the most mouthwatering scenario is hands-on impedance plethysmography, for which Jodie and Jessica strap you spread-eagle to a vertical table, turn you upside down to drain most of the blood from your legs, then measure how quickly circulation returns to normal after you've been rotated upright. (For charts and illustrations, see pages 272–275 of *The Mayo Clinic Heart Book*.) After that, since you're never too young for a physical, Jodie and I could do Jessica. Then Jodie would get her comeuppance, but good. Then it would be my turn again. Because if everyone deeply respects Doctors Without Borders (unless they make contraceptives available), what about this righteous pair of CES's Sans Merci, these Technicians Without Inhibitions?

To answer such questions, Mistress Jodie wraps a blood pressure cuff around my left biceps and pumps it up tight. Extra tight? I can't say. But it's tight. She reaches down, presses a button, and the rubber conveyor starts moving. Once I've stepped onto it, she slides her cold stethoscope under the cuff and looks at her watch. The patient is under her diagnostic, diabolical spell.

The pace at Stage 1 is a walk in the park. While Mistress Jessica monitors the long sheet of graph paper printing out my EKG pattern, Mistress Jodie points to a chart on the wall and orders me to identify my current level of stress. I'm to choose a number between 7 and 20 on the Borg Perceived Exertion Scale, with 7 being "very, very light," 13 "somewhat hard," 17 "very hard," and 20 "very, very hard."

"What about 0 through 6?" I dare ask. "Is that for 'asleep' or 'in coma'?"

Not even the ghost of an indulgent smile from the sleek dominatrix. "One is how much exertion it takes to sit back in a comfortable chair."

"Oh no, not the big, comfy chair!"

She points to the wall again. "Please pick a number."

"Okay, 7."

She nods, writes the number—efficient, impatient, in charge. It must be the AC or all these electro-suckers tugging on my flesh, but my nipples are hard. I can't help it.

"So far, so good," reports Jessica.

Adds Jodie, "We're looking for any abnormalities or ischemias."

I inhale. "Same here." I exhale. "Trying not to exhibit either one . . ."

Again, she looks peeved. She also looks good when she's peeved, as Mayo dominatrixes must. But what if I had a heart attack right here and now, Nelson Rockefeller–style? I've heard this occurs in three of every ten thousand stress tests, though what better place to have one, if have one you must? Jodie would perform mouth-to-mouth while Jessica, well, while Jessica "manned the EKG." 'Cause you know how we do, Roc-A-Fella, fo-eva . . .

Three minutes into the test, Jodie presses a button: the incline becomes twice as steep, and the treadmill speeds up. Quite a lot. So much so, in fact, that it's hard to keep my balance on the thing. When I put my right hand on the wooden support bar, Jodie instructs me, "Don't touch that." This even though the veneer has worn through in two hand-size places, presumably from *being touched.* Has she chosen an extra-strict application of the protocol for her favorite disobedient patient? Because he's displeased her somehow? The idea inspires a new burst of energy. *¡Andale!*

"If necessary," she softens, "you can balance yourself with one finger." She also encourages me to tell her when I want to stop. "Especially if you have any chest pain, or you're just out of gas."

Yes, Mistress Jodie. I'm panting a little by now, but I certainly don't want to stop, even though the Bruce protocol apparently calls for neither impedance plethysmography nor the fitting of a large Foley catheter.

"How hard is it now?"

"Huh, 'somewhat hard,' huh, I would say." But I wish she hadn't said out of *gas*, since the results of the colonoscopy haven't entirely dissipated.

"Thirteen or fourteen?"

"Fourteen, huh," I gasp, clenching my buttocks while huffing and straining not to get whipped backwards off the conveyor. "Hard-huh-minus."

She nods, writes the number. If this were my usual regimen, namely pedaling bicycle-style, I know I'd be doing much better. I'm spending too much concentration and energy just keeping my balance and responding to my mistress's cool interrogatives. Then she smiles, though just barely, and I pump a tad harder.

By the time she makes the climb faster and steeper a third time, I'm definitely puffing and sweating. And thirsty. Hensrud told me yesterday that if you have the stress test after the colonoscopy, there's a risk of becoming dehydrated. "If any problems come up with dehydration or feeling light-headed," he promised, "they'll stop the test. You just tell them." But I don't want to wimp out for Jodie. After a couple more minutes of this, however, I'm forced to admit, "I'm at 18 or 19." I stupidly put up my hand.

"Stop?" Jodie asks.

Regretting it already, I nod, and she turns off the treadmill. Catching, or at least chasing, my breath, I'm relieved, in a way, that it's over—till I hear I lasted just nine minutes and thirty-six seconds. "This translates into a 92 percent functional capacity.

Your heart rate rose from 56 to 163, your blood pressure from 102/64 to 168/80."

Knowing I got off her machine prematurely, my heart sinks, skips a beat, topples sideways. Then it starts gyrating spastically. Because first one by one, then six or eight at a time, Jodie is yanking the archipelago of electrodes from my torso, *pop-pop-pop-pop-pop-pop*, causing fifteen separate plus-minus dopamine rushes to fire simultaneously in the anterior cingulate of my frontal cortex, and my mouth to blurt, *"Hunh! Hunh!* . . . Uh, uh, really," I say, recovering a shred of composure. "I could've done more. A lot more. At *least* another twenty-four seconds." I was *far* from completely fatigued: no symptoms of exhaustion, no gasping or trembling. I simply had nothing recent to compare a 19 against. Just because I almost never pushed myself that far in real life didn't mean I couldn't push farther. I'd actually been at 16 or 17 . . .

"You can put on your shirt now," says Jessica.

When I keep on insisting "I coulda nailed ten minutes easy, without any problem at all," and thus achieved normalcy, Jessica nods. Jodie shrugs. Even James Gandolfini's charms would be lost on these two, I decide. Unless the idea of contradictory signifieds is what triggered that wicked if brief little glint I caught in Jodie's eye while she counted my pulses . . .

"You did fine, Mr. McManus," she says. "Really. Just fine. Dr. Gau will explain all the numbers."

Gerald Gau is tallish, not lean, with gray hair and beard bracketing healthy pink cheeks. Haberdasherywise, he's as tweedy as they come, a regular old-school professor, which in fact is what he is. (Me too, as it happens, though a little less tweedy most days.) As

I sit on his couch, afternoon sunlight blasts from behind him through what must be a south-facing window.

Armed with my stress test and other results, Gau shows me a chart of nonmodifiable risk factors: Personal History of Heart Attack, Bypass, or Angioplasty. Family History of Heart Attack, Bypass, or Angioplasty. My resting EKG was normal, he says, as was my exercise EKG, though his voice is abnormally stern. He directs my attention to what the chart calls modifiable risk factors. My Bruce treadmill time of 9.6 minutes, for example, puts me at the fifty-sixth percentile. "This indicates moderate deconditioning," says Gau, and I cuss myself out yet again for not having pushed it for another half minute. Even more depressing is the body fat number: 26.6 fucking percent, making me more roly-poly than two thirds of men at age fifty. Small consolation that my total cholesterol, 165 mg/dl, puts me in the top 3 percent, since in boxers I'm still reminiscent of the Pillsbury Doughboy. With my good HDL at 34 mg/dl, the total/HDL ratio is 4.9, which puts me in the top 36 percent. My resting blood pressure is 102 systolic/64 diastolic, which lands me in the very top percentile. Not bad, huh?

"Your LDL we can't measure," Gau thunders quietly, tapping my 462 mg/dl triglyceride level with the lead of his pencil. "This number here wipes it out." He explains that milligrams per deciliter is the amount present in a tenth of a liter of blood—"about half a cup." His helpful conversion flashes me back to the shot glasses brimming with warm, fatty cow blood that my father, after carving the Sunday roast—while his mother, Grandma Grace, looked on, beaming—would bestow on whichever of his children had pulled off something noteworthy the previous week. Yes, indeed!

When Grandma Grace was bangin', Mae West's zaftig hourglass was the desirable figure. Nearly all men agreed when she drawled, "Too much of a good thing is wonderful." Then, having raised two fatherless boys during the Depression, Grandma Grace was even more inclined to take extra flesh as a sign of prosperity and good health. Working as a stenographer at Fordham University, she provided her sons with food, clothes, a decent apartment, and sixteen years each of Jesuit education. During the postwar economic boom, her impressive ability to get enough food on the table devolved—and was mistranslated by her younger son and my mother in a pattern repeated by millions of others in the Greatest Generation—into *more than enough*. The year I turned eight, Grandma Grace moved in with us, which gave her a chance to affectionately pour whole cream over my farina and Corn Flakes every morning, instead of just during summer and holiday visits. She plied me with Hershey bars after lunch and golden-skinned egg custards for dessert; before settling in with Jack Paar, she'd invite me to pick through her sampler for something with white cream or caramel. I won't presume to speak for my siblings, but my personal sweet tooth came in long before my back molars did. Given that I was also subjected to my parents' lavishly funded Irish Cave Man diet, it was hard to avoid getting hooked on animal protein, potatoes, white flour, sugary "treats," and any other blessed thing guaranteed to cause hypertriglyceridemia. (My taste for alcohol, which I'll talk about later, came from both sides of the family.) Everyone meant well, of course, but it doesn't change the fact that if I die, as I almost certainly will, before my threescore and ten, it will be pretty much thanks to my clueless *but affectionate* dieticians, plus Grandpa Jim's cardiovascular genes. It certainly won't be *my* fault. Why, heaven forbid!

Oh, boo-hoo-hoo-hoo-hoo, sniffle-sniffle. Poor Jimmy! His life is so short and so difficult! Too much candy and sirloin and love! Where was coolly withholding Peggy Menzel when he needed her!? And why did he have to be raised in such a prosperous country and decade?! Boo-hoo-hoo-hoo-hoo-hoo!

Like everyone else's, my sweet tooth is part of the network of neural pathways that shape, and sensors that monitor, appetite. These networks get wired long before we start making major dietary decisions for ourselves. Neurologists have yet to figure out exactly how they work, but it's clear that old eating habits die hard, and that millions and millions of baby boomers are committing, in the innocence of their enlarged hearts, what amounts to slow-motion suicide.

Among other bad things, habitual overeating stimulates the pancreas to secrete too much insulin. The liver begins to read extra insulin as a signal to release more fats (triglycerides) into our bloodstream. All these triglycerides overload fat cells, where they're supposed to be stored for the energy we'll need later on. If we don't spend the energy and refuse to stop eating, the extra fat bungs up our blood vessels.

A bare cupboard is one form of victual restraint, but appetite is tougher to rein in when affluence makes so much tasty food so effortlessly available. It used to require some physical work to put food on the table; we scythed and milled wheat, dug up root vegetables, chased turkeys and chopped off their heads. Before humans discovered agriculture about ten thousand years ago, a body's capacity to survive on fruits, nuts, and tubers was a gigantic genetic advantage, so that trait was bred into the population. Those who learned to hunt for the lean meat of game did even better. When farmers began producing cereals and dairy cattle, life got much easier but also more dangerous for the health of our cardiovascular systems, he typed while sitting on his ass for the umpteenth consecutive hour. We're descended from people who survived famines only because their bodies used fat efficiently. Those of us best equipped genetically to survive a food shortage suffer the most now that rich, tasty food is cheap and plentiful.

Two or three generations ago, even most nonfarmers got plenty of on-the-job exercise—splitting rails, forging steel, hustling to (or at) work. All that changed in the last fifty years, and it's taking us a while to recognize and deal with the consequences. What we recently saw as the luxury of driving to a climate-controlled office or supermarket, for example, is now understood to be lethal.

Some people stay leaner than others, of course. They never develop a sweet tooth, they demonstrate mouthly discipline, or they simply burn hotter—have a higher nonexercise activity thermogenesis (NEAT). Even sitting in a cubicle, they tap their feet, fidget, work to maintain erect posture. But for most of us lower-NEAT pork bellies, the older and more deskbound we become, the more sluggish the mechanisms controlling our appetite. We get what are called the diseases of affluence—obesity, diabetes, cardiovascular breakdown—although working-class folks patronizing inexpensive fast-food emporia get more than their share of such maladies. Even below the poverty line, Americans find it terribly easy to round up a surplus of calories.

These days about a quarter of us die because of a sedentary lifestyle. If the trend continues, half of us will be obese or dead by 2030, and virtually all of us will be overweight. If it hasn't already, obesity is about to overtake smoking as our deadliest controllable risk factor. Whatever the relative order of lethality, blubber and tobacco kill more of us every few minutes than bin Laden and his ilk ever will.

"Levels of 500 or higher," Gau is telling me, "are directly related to an increased risk of cardiovascular disease." At 462, I fall perilously near the top of the "moderately high" level (200–500 mg/dl), "where the risks become slightly less definite. Some studies show people with moderate levels to be at increased risk; others find no such relationship. It *appears* that elevated triglycerides are not as important a risk factor as cholesterol, but I feel it's prudent to keep triglycerides under control."

In yet another moment of cardiovascular weakness, I blurt, "What about more medication?"

Gau glares across at me in a way that commands unsmiling eye contact in return. "You'd be playing Russian roulette, taking one or two drugs every morning to lower your levels, and another drug, alcohol, at night, which would raise them." He doesn't quite grab me and bellow, "Stop drinking, moron!" or even hiss, "Cut back dramatically," but his tone makes it obvious that my drinking habits remind him of Falstaff's or, worse, Dylan Thomas's. To illustrate, he draws a seesaw with "HDL" on the lower end, "TRIG" on the higher. With an arrow going up from HDL and another descending from TRIG, he marks the directions he wants me to go. Below this he sketches an artery: two parallel arcs with an oval connecting them at one end, for a 3-D effect. (As a draftsman, he doesn't lack talent.) Inside, top and bottom, are deposits of cholesterol, marked CHO. Next he draws an HDL cholesterol guy who looks much like Pac-Man. Hungrily scarfing up bad CHO, his eye and his little mouth kill me.

The crotchety artist wants my CHO/LDL ratio below 4.0

ASAP! To get there, four things are imperative. I need to (1) elevate and maintain my heart rate between 120 and 130 for forty minutes at least five days a week. To gauge this level of exertion without wearing a pulse monitor, I should push myself to 13 or 14 on the Borg scale, "until it's somewhat hard to talk." (2) Reach and maintain my ideal weight, around 165. (3) Lower my sugar intake, and thus my triglycerides. (4) No more smoking *whatsofuckingever!* If and only if disciplined obeisance to this regimen fails to get me below 4.0 would Gau even *pretend* to consider prescribing Niaspan (time-release niacin) to go with the Zocor. Amen.

The final modifiable risk factor on his chart is Level of Stress, which he asks me to rate between 0 and 10.

"Oh, I don't know . . ." The last two times I was asked to rate stress, the options were 0–5 and 7–20, so I'm stumped for a moment. "Seven or eight," I say finally.

Gau draws a circle between those two numbers. "Why here?"

Since he asked, I give him an abridged litany of my obligations and sorrows, concluding with the death of my son. Gau tells me he's sorry, of course, but his tweedy rectitude slumps a lot more than I expected. He no longer seems to be futilely counseling a degenerate gambler and boozehound. "See that painting behind you?" he asks. I turn around to my left and look up. On the wall above the couch is a darkly pointillist canvas, maybe three feet by two, of a moth or butterfly set against a blue-black constellation painted much the same way Georges Seurat, the *Grande Jatte* guy, would depict outer space. I noticed it before I sat down, but now it is staring me in the face as Gau tells me that eleven years ago his twenty-three-year-old son, Matthew, was killed in a motor vehicle accident. We exhale and look at each other. No tears yet. No glisten. We're cowboys.

Unable to mingle with his family and other mourners at the memorial service, Gau retreated out back to his deck. "I didn't know whether I'd ever talk again." As he stared at the darkness, heartblasted, numb beyond words, an enormous red moth fluttered up and landed on the railing, slowly opening and closing its four massive wings; altogether, their span was easily that of Gau's two open hands. No moth remotely that size is native to southern Minnesota, so where had it come from? Even stranger, it did not fly away, even when Gau ducked inside for his camera and photographed it, using a flash. He now claims it stayed on his deck, or close by, for almost three hours—until the memorial for Matthew was over. As if to prove this hard-to-believe assertion, he reaches around me, takes the painting off the wall, hands it to me, keeps on talking. The moth's four wings are tan, gray, and deep brownish red. Each smaller hind wing has a pattern that resembles an eye. It's exquisite.

"Life-size," says Gau, "give or take."

"When did you paint it?"

"I didn't."

Turns out his other son, Tom, had an especially difficult time dealing with Matthew's death; to his father's professional eye, Tom even seemed to be moving toward clinical depression. Gau finally got the idea to show him the photograph he'd taken of the moth, and to tell him the story of how it hung around during the service for Matthew. Tom was a painter, after all, and he often expressed his emotions on paper and canvas. After angrily throwing out several false starts, he came up with the image I'm balancing now on my lap. "That's a robin moth," Gau continues, "and its usual range is down in Kentucky." We sit there and think about that. "Tom shows it flying off, back out into the firmament. He finally got some relief, or release, when he finished it."

"Wow."

I go on to tell him what I know of James's death, how I felt, how I feel, and what I will never find out. About pharmaceutical companies doctoring data about teens taking antidepressants. Our desperate efforts to get the most effective medication into his system, and it turns out that we and his doctors may have been poisoning him instead. James tried to kill himself at least five times: twice by hanging, once by jumping from the roof of a six-story building, crippling him and making him much more depressed.

Gau never says wow, but he nods, shakes his head. My cardio consult is over.

What a word, I keep thinking: the *firmament*. The extent of the physical universe. Where James is?

I sob.

The light in the room has started to fade by the time Gau has finished with me, and we hug. We actually hug pretty hard.

A FOOT AND A HALF
IN THE GRAVE

Who knows? If I had stopped smoking, would I have become the
strong, ideal man I expected to be?

—ITALO CALVINO, *Zeno's Conscience*

Ain't no stoppin the champagne from poppin
the drawers from droppin, the law from watchin, I hate em . . .

—JAY-Z, "Politics as Usual"

N ot long ago, *The New Yorker* ran a Michael Maslin cartoon in which a middle-aged male patient sits up appre-
hensively on the examination table. Holding his chart,
the doctor, with a serious look on his face, says, "You've got one
foot in the grave. Further testing will determine if it's your left or
your right." Even without further testing, or obeying Dr. Gau to
the letter, I clearly need to do a serious cost-benefit analysis of my
pleasures—come up with a calculus of their ramifications for my
health and actuarial span: how much fun I want to have versus
how long I want to live. There's really nothing funny about it.

Baby boomers like me have more health information by far than any generation in history; what we need is the will, or the habits of mind, to deploy it. Part of the problem, in my case at least, is that my Pleistocene brain isn't used to having Borg Perceived Exertion Scales and steep J-shaped curves against which to balance my every last soupçon of pleasure. I was raised on processed sugar, starchy carbohydrates, and the milk and flesh of animals. When I was smoking dope and storming the ramparts in college, nobody taught me how to read fractionated lipid and cholesterol panels. *So it isn't my fault, man!* No doubt mixing cigarettes and crunk juice with a triglyceride level of 462 will kill me much sooner than later, but what about *one* little Parliament Light filtered a neat, clean quarter inch away from my lips? What if I got my triglycerides down to, say, 317, and quit smoking altogether—could I then safely drink 3.7 martinis per weekend? What about per week, then? Yet what would be the point in drinking them if I couldn't also smoke a couple of cigs? Likewise, if an X ray is just as dangerous as six months braving Chicago traffic or playing poker in a California earthquake zone, do I move up to Rochester but skip future heart scans and tournaments?

My favorite, most effective aphrodisiacs are alcohol and marijuana, but even small amounts of booze will elevate triglyceride levels. I'm also aware that alcohol destroys a vital enzyme necessary for muscle contraction. Low-to-moderate doses cause blood vessels within muscles to constrict, while causing those at the surface of the skin to dilate. When blood can't reach muscles, performance is diminished. 'Nough said.

What about just getting stoned? No calories, no blood sugar issues, makes me feel even better than booze does, makes sex even sexier. And if you've wondered as I have how pot works its magic, by far the best explanation I've read (of this and a dozen other mysteries) is in Michael Pollan's *Botany of Desire*. "The THC in marijuana and the brain's endogenous cannabinoids work in much the same way," he writes, "but THC is far stronger and more persistent than anandamide, which, like most neurotransmitters, is designed to break down very soon after its release . . . What this suggests is that smoking marijuana may overstimulate the brain's built-in forgetting faculty, exaggerating its normal operations. [And] it is the relentless moment-by-moment forgetting . . . that gives the experience of consciousness under marijuana its peculiar texture . . . Common foods taste better, familiar music is suddenly sublime, sexual touch revelatory." By momentarily forgetting how wonderful sex always is, we see, hear, and taste things "with a new keenness, as if with fresh eyes and ears and taste buds."

My almost four decades of landmark investigations have shown that smoking marijuana intensifies sexual pleasure by an average factor of 4.87. According to Murray Mittleman, a professor at the Harvard School of Public Health, it also makes you five times more prone to a myocardial infarction. Smoking pot, he says, "causes the heart rate to increase by about forty beats a minute" during the first hour. "Blood pressure increases, then abruptly falls when the person stands up. This could precipitate a heart attack." So just don't stand up, right? No problem. But neither can I forget that smoking pot is nearly twice as dangerous as vigorous lovemaking; for some folks, combining the two is almost a recipe for suicide. On the other hand, orgasms head off prostate cancer . . .

In his great book *The Denial of Death* (1973), completed just before he died of colon cancer at forty-nine, Ernest Becker described our struggle to maintain what he called the proper doses of experience. There are points of diminishing returns, he believed, beyond which we are "not helped by more 'knowing,' but only by living and doing in a partly self-forgetful way. As Goethe put it, we must plunge into experience and then reflect on the meaning of it. All reflection and no plunging drives us mad; all plunging and no reflection, and we are brutes." Each brutish ejaculation, however, each drag off a spliff or a cigarette, each mouthful of garlic mashed potatoes or Billecart-Salmon brut rosé deducts x minutes, y seconds (or x hours, y minutes) from what any competent actuary would divine is the span of my life. If I want to partake of these pleasures, I need to be willing to give up, oh, say, a windy Saturday afternoon during which one of my daughters might speak as valedictorian of her law school class, get married, score her first goal, have a daughter or son of her own, or graduate from junior kindergarten. For each cigarette. For each swallow. For each scrumptious bite. That's the deal. Yet I don't want to serve out my days in a sterile pod sucking on low-carb stones while I wait for the good stuff to happen; I need to live large! (But not chubby.) What I crave, bottom line, is the maximum number of primo life units, all told.

I'm reasonably confident I can forgo the butts and the hard stuff for the rest of my days; there will always be Heaven, after all, in which to smoke an infinity of Marlboro Reds while slurping my googolplexth Grey Goose martini. (If my mom still insists there's a Heaven, there *must* be a Heaven. Right? Right.) In the meantime, here on earth, I'll tender my resignation from the Heavy Fuel Crew, start spending more time at the gym and the farmers' market with Jennifer. *Honey, don't these pink radish sprouts look positively mouthwatering?* But stop drinking wine? One of the most beautiful things human beings have ever created? That's a trade-off I don't wanna make. Yet my calculus is bellowing at me that even if drinking moderate amounts of red wine works as part of a heart-healthy regimen, people with lofty triglycerides need to do without it entirely . . .

Aaaaaaaaaaaaaaaaaaaaaaaaaaaaaaaaaaaaaaaaaaaaaaaaaaaaaaaaaaa-aaaaaaaaaaaaaaaaaaaaaaaaaaaaaaaaaaaaaaaaaaaaaaaaaaaaaaaaaaaaaa-aaaaaaaaaaaaaaaaaaaaaaaaaaaaaaaaaaaaaaaaaaaaaaaaaaaaaaaaaaaaaa-aaaaaaaaaaaaaaaaaaaaaaaaaaaaaaaaaaaaaaaaaaaaaaaaaaaaaaaaaaaa-aaahhhh!!!!

So, said the calculating self-medicator. Now we can get down to business.

Stomach full, pupils dilated at 8 a.m. Wednesday, I listen to Douglas Cameron's brief lecture on floaters and flashes, unable for the moment to read the six-page handout from the American Academy of Ophthalmology. Blind to print—wow, what a nightmare!

I ask Dr. Cameron whether, to preserve my eyesight, I should read less and, even scarier, write less.

"Your eyes work just as hard when you're reading as when you're staring into space," Cameron is happy to tell me. "Lids shut or open, the eye doesn't know the difference. What gets tired when you have to concentrate for a while is the blinking muscle. The reason it feels like we get 'eye headaches' is that there are so many sensitive nerves surrounding, but not actually part of, the eye. To preserve your eyesight, you should exercise, eat right, not smoke."

I tell him that for the last two days I've been trying to decide whether to stop drinking altogether, since I've never been good at taking moderate doses of booze, food, cigarettes—for that matter, anything. As we continue with my exam, Cameron (who resembles a younger Tom Brokaw) loosens up enough to admit that he's more dyslipidemic than I am. "But still, I drink wine every night." I'm even more thrilled to hear that his cardiologist is Gau, and that our esteemed mutual physician just got back from a cook's tour of France, where he gave free rein to his connoisseur's appetite for that country's gastronomic and viticultural abundance. Cameron insists more than once that he's *not* recommending his own behavior, or even Dr. Gau's. As an M.D., he's capable of making "a highly informed decision" for himself, not for me, on these matters.

"But how many glasses a night?" I must know.

"Oh, two or three, sometimes four or five . . ."

"Red or white are we talking? I've heard red is healthier, heartwise."

"Depends on what's for dinner." He shrugs. "Mostly red, though." He frowns. "Don't tell Gau."

Tell Gau? Not on your life, O my brother! But I'll certainly make a note to weigh all these facts in my calculus. In the meantime, Douglas Cameron for Chief Medical Officer of the Mayo Clinic! Douglas Cameron for King of the World!

My dermatologist, Wendy Wu, is tall for an Asian woman, with crow-black hair and protuberant cheekbones. Her female intern sports heply rectangular specs on diligent, wide hazel eyes. Both doctors are friendly enough, though it quickly begins to seem that they see me as an executive cadaver of sorts, to be fingered and diced for the sake of the intern's education. What I thought were a few nothing freckles and warts, for example, Dr. Wu identifies for her student as "several lesions on his anterior right shin," though she does note that I have "no personal or family history of skin cancers, including melanoma." More specifically, I have "a mild to moderate amount of sun damage." Next she identifies "several pigmented lentigines. Also set on his central forehead is an ill-defined hyperkeratotic erythematous papule with some pigment in it," not exactly the way my crack team of publicists would phrase it. "*Hyperkeratotic*," says Wu when I ask, "means thickened skin, and *erythematous* means red. Papules are small, inflamed swellings that don't produce pus." No translation required to gather "some greasy yellowish scaliness visible" on my scalp doesn't mean chick magnet, probably.

Worse, what I thought was a slow-to-heal bug bite on my right shin is actually "an erythematous papule with a hint of telangiectasia," deemed fit by Dr. Wu for a biopsy. "And superior to this is a hyperkeratotic stuck-on-appearing papule against an erythematous background." Her plan of attack? Liquid nitrogen, one squirt per papule. To Wu's eye, the papule farther down my shin looks even more ominous—"suspicious for a superficial basal cell carcinoma versus hypertrophic actinic keratosis versus squamous cell carcinoma." She orally obtains my informed consent for a "shave biopsy." Now? "Yes, right now. My intern can do it." She can?

The intern, who suddenly looks seventeen and is wearing, I can't help but notice, the same glasses *art* students favor, warns me "the local will burn a little" just before injecting me with lidocaine and epinephrine. It does. As Wu looks on with a cool, narrow eye, the intern daubs me again with alcohol, shaves a few hairs, writes something in her notebook, and begins hacking away at my shin with a mean-looking grater, as though preparing to make a cheese omelet or assist in a Kinsey experiment. In the meantime, Wu has turned her attention to a pair of tiny moles on my forehead, freezing them with a kind of fizzy dry ice sprayed from an aerosol canister. *Zzzt! Zzzt! Zzzt!* Ow! *Magister mullia sapiens—NOT!*

"You should have these watched, Mr. McManus." *Zzzt! Zzzt!* Ow! Shit! "I wu, Dr. Will. I mean, I will."

"What?" *Zzzt!*

"I will! Yes! I . . ."—this as a bandage is being taped to my shin—"but" *Zzzt!* "how many more . . ."

Back down the elevator, finally, and into a gleaming subway teeming with blind people, burn victims, hairless seven-year-olds, he-men on crutches, older folks twisted in wheelchairs . . . and me navigating among them, if barely, what with my bandaged shin, my frozen warts, my blurred vision, my warring selves, my hypertriglyceridemia.

Feel sorry for yourself much, you fortunate candyass motherfucker?

Can't help it. My shin hurts. My forehead—

His shin hurts. Why don't you take a peek at all of these—

Can't really see them.

You see them.

Plus I've got this fatty plaque clogging my arteries, calcifying away as we speak.

You do?

Yeah. Gonna kill me.

How soon?

We're gonna find *out* now how soon, motherfucker.

Nine-fifty-nine a.m., one minute early for my fateful "chest CT without biopsy" at Rochester Methodist's Department of Diagnostic Radiology. I'm ushered in right away and introduced to a technician, who positions me faceup on a gray padded plank. Instead of standing with my chest (or back, or side) against an X-ray plate to produce a single 2-D image, I lie on the plank with my hands above my head as the machine slides me through the round hole of a square X-ray doughnut. Whirring and clicking, the gantry rotates around my chest, zapping me with invisible somethings while the opposite surface detects how much radiation makes it through the arteries in my chest. Inside the doughnut's big brain, numeric values have been programmed to generate what would otherwise be a blur into a clear three-dimensional cross section of my coronary arteries. Since calcified plaque is too hard for X rays to penetrate, it shows up pale gray, much like bone, on the negative. Within the next twenty-four hours, a cardiac radiologist will read between the lines of this picture.

For my final debriefing, Hensrud and I sit side by side reading Gau's verdict: "If his coronary calcium scan shows that he is greater than seventy-fifth percentile for his age, I would aggressively urge stopping all alcohol and going ahead with the niacin in any case. I would be more assertive"—*even more* assertive, he should say—"if the progression of his scan indicates that he is getting a more rapid progression of his atherosclerotic process."

When a cardiocowboy with Gau's credentials uses language like this, only an obstinate moron refuses to heed him. Hensrud, the good cop, agrees—to a point. "The less alcohol the better when it comes to triglycerides. But at this point, giving up wine may not be realistic for you. To get maximum cardiovascular benefit, Dr. Gau gave you a heart rate to shoot for which will give you the most bang for your buck in terms of your arteries." Translation: my cardiovascular profile should not inspire oodles of confidence, but nor am I ready for AA or open-heart surgery. Depending on what the scan shows, I'll be permitted a glass or two of pinot gris with my trout of an evening, or not; too much new calcification and I'll be quaffing Volvic and Niaspan for the rest of my days, and there may not be many more *of* them. But Hensrud is willing to wait for the "final final" decision on wine until the results of the heart scan come in. "Probably later today, after you leave. But I'll call you. Maybe not till tomorrow, however." So be it.

Where the e-form asks for a general impression of the patient, Hensrud typed: "Slightly overweight, pleasant, and straightforward male." Whatever *straightforward* means, I love the way *slightly* repudiates that sixty-seventh-percentile bullshit on Gau's body-fat scale, which has got to be off. It's just *got* to! Jessica must have miscalibrated my love handle, and I'd like to barge back into her dungeon, demand a kinder and gentler recaliperization, then give her a "somewhat hard" spanking. "Didn't you hear Dr. Hensrud?" *Whack! Whack!* "I'm slightly! Plus for your information," *smack-smack-smack*, "I am *pleasant!*"

She may also be interested to know that the following parts of me have been Mayofficially deemed "normal or unremarkable": abdomen, chest, ears, nose, throat, extremities, gait, genitalia (not unhealthily huge, thank the Lord), head, joints, lungs, lymph, mental, neuro, rectum, spine, thyroid, and vessels. My diverticulitis has healed, though the biopsy of my mole is still pending. The one performed by Dr. Susan Abraham revealed my polyp to be "a granular tissue, inflammatory polyp," says Hensrud. "Not cancerous, in other words. Not precancerous, either. You can therefore wait at least five years until your next colonoscopy."

"By which point the Fleet prep will have been upgraded to three flutes of vintage Cristal."

"One flute, in your case."

"Even so, I can't wait."

The trip home lasts less than six hours. I'm pooped and my pupils are dilated, so Jennifer drives the whole way. Our daughters are mesmerized by the gauze on my shin oozing blood, as well as the pair of scarlet boo-boos adorning my forehead, and they want explanations. But what can I say? Daddy's not only been reamed, steamed, and dry-cleaned, he's been bled, scraped, shaved, freeze-dried, stressed, scanned, and sanded, all by the best in the business.

"Why?"

"Because Daddy wants to be here to answer your questions for as long as humanly possible."

"Why?"

"Actually," says Jennifer, "he doesn't wanna be here quite *that* long."

"But where is he *going?*" asks Beatrice.

We arrive home to seventeen voicemails, but I really only care about one. "Mr. McManus, hi, this is Dr. Hensrud from Mayo."

Gulping and suddenly thirsty, I sit at the dining room table amid five days of junk mail. If I could just find a pen, I could write what he says on the back of our gas bill. "Those two things we left pending: the homocysteine, which is that blood test similar to cholesterol, that was fine. There's no problem at all with that." Good, okay, swell, so which result *was* there a problem with? "The other was the coronary calcification scan"—*yeah?*—"and good news on that also. There was absolutely no new coronary calcification. Although this doesn't eliminate the possibility of any narrowing, it markedly decreases any risk of that. So that's good news!" Then he reminds me to keep taking aspirin and tells me to call him in the morning.

Jazzed to the point of Swing on the Hard Bop Continuum, I uncork Veuve Clicquot to toast this gold-plated testimony that I don't have to die, not that it was ever in doubt. *I really am bullet-proof, baby!* After two and four-sevenths flutes, however, Jennifer gives me her look. "But didn't Hensrud say that—"

"But nothing," I tell her. "*Tomorrow* I'll get with the new Spartan regimen."

"Now Jimmy, you promised us. You've been swearing all day up and down."

"Slainte!"

Two weeks later the bill comes: $8,484.25. *Harper's* pays it, though not everyone's happy about it, mainly because we'd been told that executive physicals typically run between three and four grand. When I call the billing office and then Dr. Hensrud to discuss it, the latter reminds me that the single biggest cost was the colonoscopy, and I won't need another one for quite a long time. The standard of care as recently as 1997 called for stool samples and a flexible sigmoidoscopy (an exam of the lower third of the colon), but this regimen was missing 25 percent of cancers and other health problems. Now a colonoscopy is the gold standard. Since it's more effective in preventing cancer, it's vastly less expensive in the long run, even though the initial bill may seem on the high side.

Hensrud also tells me that whatever money the Executive Program nets from the $250 fee circulates back into the general budget to cover Medicare patients, for whom the government reimburses Mayo only thirty cents on the dollar. "These costs have to be made up somewhere," he says, then reminds me that many executive patients make charitable contributions on top of paying their bill out of pocket. The clinic's relationship with such patients is critical not only to its operating budget, but to everyone's health care. Shiny, happy donors give more for medical research.

Johns Hopkins and the Cleveland Clinic have similar programs, I know, and others are springing up quickly, all designed to help institutions protect their most valuable human resources, and hospitals their bottom line. Some folks are more crucial to the success of an operation: the dean or the closer, for example, versus the teaching assistant or the guy hawking peanuts. This *isn't* to say teaching assistants or food vendors should receive lower-quality or less compassionate treatment if they become sick or injured, only that we monitor the wellness of more senior or less replaceable players a bit more proactively. Such notions don't fly in some quarters, of course. Americans think it's okay to sell Porsches and Pontiacs, and we understand that Scott Turow can't appeal everyone's death sentence. With health care, we aren't so sure.

Hensrud points to key differences between his program and what he calls concierge services. He doesn't offer (or charge for) around-the-clock cell-phone access. He makes no house calls. He provides no luxurious accommodations, unless you count the little refrigerator in the lounge with the gratis packets of chicken goo. As employees of an emphatically not-for-profit clinic, he and his colleagues are determined to strike a balance between a bare-bones approach that might miss something fatal and boutiques that do full body scans and make house calls for anyone who pays the steep fee. Regardless of income or insurance, everyone who comes through the door of the Mayo Clinic gets the same basic preventive services, the same amount of time with doctors who have the same diagnostic acumen. "The target metrics of the executive program are exactly the same as the others," Hensrud says. "The same number of RVUs [relative value units] are apportioned for every exam. We need to be cost effective, and by that I mean reasonable yet thorough. Everyone gets a urinalysis because they're cheap, for example, but also because they tell us a lot." My $400 consult with Gau and the $540 heart scan were clinically indicated by Hensrud's reading of my test results, and the $3,200 colonoscopy was standard for someone my age, but *any* patient with similar numbers would be seen by a Szarka or a Gau or an equally capable specialist. Hensrud regrets that it's harder of late to schedule a routine wellness checkup at Mayo, but the reason for that isn't money. "Our traditional mission as a tertiary referral center"—that is, as the clinic of last resort for patients whose symptoms have baffled the rest of the medical community—"is a service we need to provide for more people, irrespective of their ability to pay for it. There's only so many staff, so many square feet . . ."

The previous April, five Democratic members of Congress— including Illinois senator Richard Durbin—urged President Bush to review the legality of boutique practice charging membership fees while billing Medicare. Also weighing in on boutique ethics was William Petasnick, CEO of Froedtert Memorial Lutheran Hospital. Petasnick says the boutiques threaten to pull the most profitable patients (mainly, those who can afford elective surgery) from urban acute-care teaching hospitals, which will soon be less able to "underwrite community-based services"—that is, to treat poor people.

Those who favor a moderated two-tier system describe it as a pragmatic return to old-fashioned medicine, in which more time is spent educating and treating patients, less time filling out forms, with a greater emphasis on prevention instead of treating health problems after it's too late. Jim Levine, a harried young primary care physician with 4,300 patients in Brookline, Massachusetts, is considering an invitation to enter a concierge practice. "If you want to solve the homeless problem," he said, "you build low-income housing. You don't stop people from buying mansions."

Others argue that instead of a multitiered system, all physicians should provide the same services to all patients, regardless of their ability to pay, and that it's unconscionable to increase the burden shouldered by the physicians who remain in the trenches. Professor John Goodson of Harvard Medical School says concierge medicine "undermines the most fundamental commitments of our profession," calling it "the Balkanization of American medicine." It's impossible to disagree with a well-intentioned expert like Goodson, but I also can't help wondering who *his* doctor is, and how long he waits to see him or her.

Concierge medicine got off the ground in Seattle in 1996, when the former team doctor of the Supersonics founded MD^2 to provide nonathletes with the caliber of medical service NBA players receive. Feel a twinge in your meniscus at 4 a.m.? Call me. I'm comin' right over.

Some programs charge $20,000 per patient per year, others as little as $900. All provide doctors with a much lighter patient load: four hundred instead of four thousand; three or four patients a day instead of two or three dozen. They offer same-day appointments, cell-phone numbers of doctors, even house calls.

Such programs have naturally come under fire. Dr. Fitzhugh Mullan says boutique medicine "represents a fracturing of the social compact where everyone is cared for under a common covenant. The whole notion of health insurance is that we have a risk pool and that when we are well, we pay into it, and we get no benefit from that. But when we are sick, we are taken care of and other people's money pays to cover our expenses." To opt out of traditional health care into a boutique practice is not "a responsible way to use one's training as a physician." We should concentrate our resources on delivering adequate care to everyone, Mullan and others believe, not on pampering the affluent. While Princeton economist Uwe Reinhardt likens American health care to a 747 with three classes of service but in which every passenger arrives at the same destination at the same time, Mullan points out that boutique patients are buying their own Lear jets and hiring the best 747 pilots to fly them.

Doctors, after all, are our last line of defense against illness and death. If the most important thing in the world is your health, then access to Mayo-caliber care is the ultimate luxury. It shouldn't be a luxury, perhaps, but it is. If we're smart, if we're lucky, such clinics will be the future of health care, as the Mayo has been since its founding 117 years ago.

As the cutting edge rips into the future, some folks will be admitted to the world's finest hospitals and others—because of geography, health insurance, the nature of their disease, the malpractice laws of their state or their country, whether or not they live in a war zone—will not. Some will be accepted by lottery, or because of the severity of their condition, into trial treatment programs; some won't. Roughly half who get in will be given placebos; sometimes the treatment the other half gets will extend their lives, sometimes it will shorten them. Many of these conundrums have less to do with social engineering than what used to be called existentialism. Some things are better worked through by advancing the state of the art, or by painting an alien moth, than by trying to rig an identical outcome for everyone.

Western medicine's war on disease will progress much more slowly, or stop, if the financial incentive is idealistically curtailed altogether: a humanitarian impulse is simply no match for a virus. Call me naive, but if the makers of statins hadn't known ahead of time they could earn a fair profit, they wouldn't have suffered the risk and expense of developing them, and lots of us dyslipidemics would be strokebound in wheelchairs, or cremated. Ditto for the makers of synthetic human insulin, AIDS vaccines, and the like. To those who could never afford these nonmiracles, drug companies should give them away, having built that cost into the prices the rest of us pay. Governments should help out with tax money, too, and fundamentalist Christians should be no more able to rein in stem-cell research or women's reproductive rights than fundamentalist Muslims are. Praise the Lord, or Allah, and pass the damn biotechnology.

PEARL JAM

When Bea spoke of having had a checkered career, she was taking a sarcastic or disparaging tone that did not reflect what she really felt about her life of love affairs. [They] were the main content of her life, and she knew that she was not being honest when she belittled them.

—ALICE MUNRO, "Vandals"

It happened years ago and in somebody else's
Dining room. Madame X begged to be relieved
Of a sexual pain that had my name

Written all over it. Those were the days . . .

—MARK STRAND, *Dark Harbor*, XXII

Like most Americans my age, I'm on my second marriage. And my last, I hope and trust. In fact, let me substitute *in* as the rosier preposition, smacking less of the stopgap. I'm also a typical baby boomer in that I got married too young the first time, to a person I wasn't all that compatible with. Jennifer made a similar blunder herself, though she stayed married for only about a year. She and her first husband didn't have a child, perhaps the main reason their divorce was so friendly. Mine, after thirteen years and two children, was more of a dirty bomb, cesium-137 sculpted around old-fashioned dynamite, perfectly designed to trigger panicked evacuation and eliminate critical infrastructure.

This time around, my wife and I are better fixed emotionally and financially, and the fact that she's fifteen years younger than me feels in sync with our sociobiological clocks. Not that I ever wanted to become a parent again when we got married in 1992. After my first wife left me for another man in 1987, not only did my penis feel like an acorn with squirrelly toothmarks, but I was almost violently committed to not making any more children with it. I already had two and neither was terribly happy, in part because Dad didn't live with them. My talented, unlucky son, James, would develop acute schizophrenia.

By the time I'd met Jennifer, in 1989, I still had hope for James, especially now that her nurturing spirit—her calm, sane, affectionate competence—had entered our lives. We took him on road trips out west, to Bulls games, to Scotland, to the Lincoln home (and golf course) in Springfield. A good deal of our social life during the winter of 1992 consisted of watching him play basketball for the seventh-grade traveling all-stars. In one fairly miraculous game, he went off for seventeen points in a six-minute quarter: five of six threes and a breakaway layup after a steal. A hundred and thirty-six points and eight steals, I silently extrapolated, in a regulation NBA game. He was thirteen years old, five feet tall, and weighed about eighty-five pounds. There were players in the league who weighed twice that, who had hair on their forearms and calves, who shaved on a regular basis. But James could hang in with these guys. More than hang in. He usually had three or four steals and was often the game's highest scorer. That spring, he and I made matching birdies across the water on the par-three fifteenth at the Peter Jans Golf Course in Evanston. He also pitched a no-hitter in Little League, worked far beyond his grade level in math, and was becoming a badass guitarist. He was bewildered and pissed about his parents' divorce but otherwise seemed happy to be alive every minute.

During his first year of high school, however, he began gradually—then suddenly—to spiral down into infernos of rage, depression, and passive-aggressive defiance. His mother and I had divorced when he was ten, and she'd remarried and had a child a few months later, repeating her pattern with me, though she and Dan separated soon after that. Our daughter, Bridget, four years older than James, would enter a similar tailspin but eventually right herself. With James, changing schools didn't work. Tough love didn't work. New guitars didn't work, since he smashed both the instruments he received as birthday and Christmas gifts. Zoloft and Paxil and Prozac and Elavil didn't work; in fact, one or more of them may have exacerbated his suicidal impulses.

Other boys with divorced parents had posters of Hendrix, Kurt Cobain, or Keith Richards on their walls, but James took these guys at their *word*.

> *I'll meet y'all in the next world, and don't be late.*
> *I love you, I'm not gonna crack, I kill you, I'm not gonna*
>   *crack . . .*
> *Can't you see, Sister Morphine, I'm tryin' to score?*

The hardcore posturing of "Voodoo Child" and *Sticky Fingers* I'd perfunctorily deployed twenty-five years earlier was now a code my son lived by—and was ready to die for. Other psychiatrists entered the picture. So did police orders, trips to emergency rooms and mental health clinics (one for two years, out of state), a psychotic twenty-eight-year-old girlfriend, and several more attempts to harm and/or kill himself. My role in his life was reduced to the desperate, humiliated wreck slumped in the corner of the ICU, the guy who pleaded with doctors, filled out insurance forms, listened to Muzak while weeping on hold, murderously disputed with claims adjusters, and reported his only son's various addresses to cops, social workers, R.N.'s. I was gonna do my damnedest to help James any way I could for as long as it took, but under no circumstances would I voluntarily subject myself to any *new* doses of such mind-bending pain, to say nothing of the infinitely more horrendous pain *he* was in. As Raymond Carver put it while dealing with the two unhappy children of his first marriage: "I'd rather take poison than go through that again."

Which would have been just fine with Jennifer. Not long after I met her, she told me she'd lost her right ovary to a dermoid cyst five years earlier. (The size of a grapefruit, with teeth, hair, and cartilage, it was probably a malformed twin that developed inside Jennifer instead of her mother—instead of a sister, a cyst.) Informed that she was infertile by her Memphis gynecologist, Jennifer began, at eighteen, to make tough psychological adjustments. Though she wasn't completely aware of it, men who didn't want children—rare beasts—became more attractive to her. To the extent that I considered getting married again, I was looking for a wife who didn't want to become a mother, almost unheard of in young heterosexual women. In no small part because of these dovetailing yens, we allowed ourselves to fall in love during a trip to Donegal in the summer of 1990.

By the time we got married two years later, Jennifer's Chicago gynecologist, Cheryl Neihaus, had performed a laparoscopy to mitigate the painful symptoms of endometriosis. It worked. An experimental NIH program at Northwestern Hospital treated her interstitial cystitis with a colposcopy, small doses of Elavil (one of the "wonder drugs" James was taking), and a fluid-intake program called Pee School. In Jennifer's case, the combination of therapies worked. The doctors also surprised us by saying that she now had "an outside but reasonable chance" to get pregnant, if that's what she wanted. She did. More than anything, as it turned out.

This bolt from the blue stunned us into vigorous debate mode for the next seven years. I was already forty-one, forty-three, forty-five, with two adolescent children whose emotional needs were almost hilariously beyond my power to satisfy. *Nuclear family*, to me, was a joke—or a sentence. With her usual patience and grace, Jennifer tried to persuade me that just because things had gone badly with my first wife "doesn't mean *we're* doomed to go there. Ya gotta have a little faith, Jimmy."

"I know that. I want to. I do. It's just that . . ." I knew she was right in my heart and my brain, though my gut had impregnable doubts. And then there was Jennifer's gut, and her health overall. Because her doctors had also informed us that the endometriosis would be further relieved—and the risks of breast and uterine cancer reduced by a hefty percentage—if Jennifer got pregnant and nursed.

The decision seemed designed by Beelzebub to remain unresolvable. But when I kvetched about my dilemma to, among countless others, U.S. poet laureate Mark Strand, who is six seven and looks like a cross between Dante and Clint Eastwood, he gazed soulfully down at Jennifer while offering to stand in for me fatherhoodwise—the laureateship came with extra responsibilities during the Kennedy and Clinton administrations—and that by itself about settled it. Without making our decision a fait accompli, Jennifer went off the Pill, cleaned up her diet, began doing yoga and taking evening primrose oil. She wanted to be healthy and ready to go "just in case" Strand or I made a move.

Now that I was Executive Vice President, Contraception Division, I requisitioned a sampler of Sagami Excaliburs, Contempo Rough Riders, Trojan Horses, and leftover Inspiral "spring action" glow-in-the-dark Christmas Specials, in flavors including Boeufsteck, Mistletoe, Kiwi, and Bubblegum Blast. We were set.

In the fall of '97, Jennifer and I spent a five-week residency at the Rockefeller Foundation's Villa Serbelloni in Bellagio, Italy. It was, in two words, kinda posh. Virgil and Catullus lovingly refer to the place, as do both Plinys, who had a summer home there, the Villa Pliniana, in the years immediately after Jesus was born. The present villa was commandeered in 1943 by the SS, who deployed it as R&R quarters for Luftwaffe pilots. Ella Walker, the whiskey heiress, had purchased it in 1928, and she refurbished it after the war. She died in 1959 having bequeathed it to the Rockefeller Foundation, whose president that year was Dean Rusk. It was Rusk who decided the villa should be used as a haven for artists, writers, and scientists.

The room Jennifer and I were assigned, No. 9, had views of both the Lecco and Como arms of the lake, and of numerous Alps. We were told that Jack Kennedy had one of his last presidential trysts in this room in June of '63, during a series of state visits to European capitals. (Mrs. Kennedy, seven months pregnant with Patrick—who would die when he was less than two days old—stayed home with five-year-old Caroline and two-year-old JFK, Jr.) An audience with the pope had been scheduled, but when John XXIII died, Kennedy had a political problem: our first Catholic president's attendance at Paul VI's ascension on June 21 might have made him appear unduly in thrall to the Vatican, as had been widely predicted during the 1960 campaign against Nixon. Rusk, now secretary of state, persuaded his boss to lie low at the Villa Serbelloni before heading to Germany, where he made his *Ich bin ein Berliner* speech on June 26.

During our own romantic interlude in Room No. 9, Jennifer and I must have had twenty-five days of brisk autumn sun, which gave first the Lecco arm a blindingly platinum glitter, and then, as we got dressed for sumptuous dinners, the Como. High in the mountains that Halloween Eve, with preposterously excellent moonlight ricocheting off the deepest freshwater in Europe, it finally sank in for me that only a bona fide fuckwad would compromise the health of his beautiful young wife while depriving her of parenthood. She had, after all, saved my life by marrying me, and I sensed that she'd make a great mother. As I performed my husbandly duty sans condom, however, I was hoping, like a bona fide fuckwad, that somehow it wouldn't quite take. Women on both sides of her family had serious fertility problems, after all, and we'd been warned by doctors that Jennifer heavy with child was a long shot. So was I bluffing or hedging my bet? Neither one. As pokeristas have it, I was betting on the come and all-in.

When a pee test said Jennifer was pregnant and her gynecologist, Brian Foley, confirmed it, I pretended to be thrilled. I even had the balls to take credit for something I'd literally prayed wouldn't happen, accepting thumbs-ups and fists from my friends and lying to my pregnant wife through the following August, when, after thirty-eight hours of labor, twenty-five on Pitocin, Beatrice was born in the middle of an emergency C-section. Her name, from Dante's great love and Jennifer's great-aunt, means "bringer of joy," and she had. When a nurse finally handed her to me under the warming lamp, I got juiced to the point of delirium. *Wham!* When you're suddenly forced to understand that one of the very best things in your life is something you've battled for years with all your guile and strength to head off, it shakes your self-confidence. In a good way, but still.

A similar bolt had struck me a couple of years after my first marriage ended very, very much against my wishes. But what if I'd had a vasectomy then, as many fathers do upon getting divorced? What if Jennifer died or left me and, after a period of mourning, I fell in love with a woman who wanted, who *needed*, to have children with me, in spite of my imminent, or in-progress, geezerhood? In my spiraling existential confusion, I decided that Jennifer and I should make another baby ASAP, and we did. The day we got green-lighted to resume "full" conjugal relations, Grace was conceived. Our Irish-twin girls, born fourteen and a half months apart, were soon insisting they needed a baby brother or sister, but so far our vizsla, Buzz Likeyear, is the best we've been able to come up with.

And now, as a fifty-plus father of four, I'm tempted to get a vasectomy. Jennifer will be fertile for another few years, though we seem to be done having children. Except for brief interludes with a diaphragm and during two pregnancies, she has been on the Pill since she was a junior in high school. Dr. Foley says that her estrogen dosage is safe, but Jennifer still has concerns about how long she's been on it. Though we both feel terribly lucky to have Dr. Foley and the rest of Western medicine at our disposal, the catastrophic error of hormone replacement therapy makes it hard to have absolute faith in the OB/GYN state of the art.

The last time I'd looked into it, a vasectomy involved my vasa deferentia—sperm ducts running from testes to penis—being severed and cauterized, something like taking a Zippo to the end of a straw. Once the sizzle and acrid black smoke abated, spermatozoa would no longer mix with the seminal fluid produced in my prostrate, as Andy Sipowicz calls it. Dammed upstream from my epididymis, they would be harmlessly reabsorbed by my body. Voilà! Sex without consequences. Plus I'd finally be shouldering the contraceptive burden for Jennifer. A no-brainer, then, I suppose . . . except that I can't help wondering which streams of my consciousness might also back up into a swamp teeming with in-bred poachers, birth-deformed human-faced reptoids, and other psychosexual quicksand. Might the damming not add yet another strangled voice, or trillions of strangled voices, to the chorus of drips already echoing in my libidinal cesspool? Wouldn't the knowledge that I'm firing blanks put a serious ding in what's left of my cowboy self-confidence? Some things you don't wanna tamper with.

From talking to doctors and Googling endless reports, I've been given to understand that 99 percent of the time, erectile function remains unimpaired following a competent vasectomy. But what about that luckless 1 percent? When half a million Americans and four million men worldwide get snipped every year, we're talking 110 new guys a *day* who can't get it up anymore, and that gives me pause.

Pause? It gives me the wifefucking willies!

Then there's the Irish Catholic ethos I was raised in—eighteen years of unrelieved balderdash about how sex without intending to conceive a child is a grave mortal sin, how left unconfessed it consigns you to Hell for eternity, and how whatever incidental pleasure you feel during procreation is pure wavy gravy. Thus, if I got a vasectomy, I'd *never* be able to make love legitimately, at least according to the most priest-ridden nooks of my conscience. And if I didn't still sorta believe these things, Grandma Grace, I probably wouldn't've named my third daughter after you. U.I.O.G.D., as you and the Sisters always made me write at the top of my homework assignments. *Ut in omnibus gaudetur Dei,* nome sayin'? That in all things God may be glorified. Sorely tempted by wanton Catholic schoolgirls exposing the backs of their knees between maroon socks and pleated plaid skirts, we were strictly limited to priest-approved pickup lines: "Excuse me, is this pew taken?" "I didn't know angels flew this low," and (from your knees) "May I drinketh from your cuppeth?" Forty years later a lap dance in the executive lounge of Spearmint Rhino will continue to be grounds for both earthly divorce and an eon or two on God's Weber. Even though substantial tracts of my brain don't believe in Him anymore, my flayed atheistic carcass will be smoking and crispy, dripping little yellow globules of fat on the coals—*pop pop pop pop*—as I rotate, imaginatively trussed like a

free-range, hundred-percent organic, freethinking chicken, on a
skewer driven up through my sweetmeats . . .

"I will not be reconstructed" was the immortal Shane
MacGowan's soberest eroto-theological dictum, back when he
was still the Pogues' front man, though he clearly needed work on
his teeth. Two of my close friends agree. "No one's goin' anywhere
near there with surgical implements," drawls my agent, hitching a
cocky thumb crotchward. My colleague Paul demands to know,
"What if, after a war or a natural calamity, I was called upon to
help repopulate the planet? Or what if all my children died, in a
plane crash, for example? What if my wife died and, after a period of mourning, I fell in love with a woman who wanted, who
needed, to have children with me?" Even in his sixties, America's
best living poet still snarls, "I'm here to create a new imperial empire; gonna do whatever circumstances require." And without
Dylan's irony, one of my poker buddies unequivocally declares:
"The folks who wanna wipe out Americans are breeding five or
six times faster than we are, so we fuckin'-A better get busy."

Because of my half-decent health and what Richard Ford might
call the ultimate good luck, I'm not yet in need of Viagra. Even
dumb-luckier, thirteen years into our till-death commitment I'm
still head over heels with my wife. Making love with her is how
our daughters were conceived, only two of the reasons I sometimes experience far more kinky *and* old-fashioned intimacy in
her moist, naked presence than I ever imagined was possible. Yet
maybe we've seen each other naked, helped each other to vomit,
handled each other's laundry a few times too often to pretend we
still reside in the Pre-Serpent Garden of Eden. Neither of our

chest-waist-hip ratios is what it used to be—mainly, in Jennifer's case, because she bore our girls into the world and then lavishly nursed them. Caesarean scars may escalate my emotional commitment, but not my libidinal interest. And I am no Daniel Day-Lewis. Which may be why Jennifer has been reading so many Munro stories.

If you still love and care about your wife but no longer lust, if you ever did, only for her a hundred percent of the time, what are the options for the Modern American Husband? Good Jim is here to tell you that the honorable course is to stay faithful to her, especially if she's the mother of your children. Keep a fifth of *anejo* in the freezer, a spliff in the drawer of your nightstand. Requisition posh lingerie, manufacture scenarios, make catholicguilt.com your home page, augment the mood with accoutrements. Liquor up front, poker in the rear, but avoid any tournaments played in Amsterdam, Paris, L.A., or Las Vegas. Hire a babysitter, but only to take care of the kids while you and their mom spend a night at the Hilton. Make do.

What about that old warhorse, honesty? Is it still the best policy, even when admitting to your wife that your lust for her may have been reduced by even a single bottom quark? When owning up to aspirations that involve other women would make her feel contemptuous of you and awful about herself? (Or, almost as bad, make her wait till you're asleep before stabbing you in the eye with a bowie knife, plunging it all the way up to the hilt, logically enough, in the eye you used to peep at a sunbathing neighbor, as a jealous wife does in Denis Johnson's classic "Emergency.") What should you do when you don't have permission to *have* these physical urges, let alone to admit them? Answer: sometimes you have to go to bed with the woman you have, not the woman you want. Because you can have all the "armor" in the world on a "tank" and it can still be "blown up." You can lead a horse to water, if you follow my drift, but you can't make it hold its nose to the grindstone. A bird in the hand beats the pants off pathetically ogling students or certified exercise specialists, so you need to make hay while you can still hit the nail on the head.

A few years ago a teaching colleague happened to share with me how he'd "totally unpushily" suggested to his wife that they "might make an interesting threesome" with the unattached red-haired woman living in the riverfront condominium two floors below theirs. The suggestion was greeted with such piercing ululations that he retracted it at once. All I meant was, etc., etc. He and his wife remain undivorced, but they also had to sell their great condo and *move*.

Bottom line? To have as my wife a beautiful woman like Jennifer, who loves me, who is the mother of our daughters and step-mother to Bridget, and who may still want to have another child with me—I cannot risk mucking this up.

No decent husband or father (or poker player) would ever admit this, but getting divorced is also impractical. No man or woman should underestimate how luxuriously *convenient* it is, as the Church Lady might say, to be married. Actuaries will attest that both you and your children will live longer, while pollsters say happier, doctors say healthier, accountants say wealthier. *Stay married or die* says the memo our culture has written. For subtler analysis, here's how Marianne Moore began what may well be her mistresspiece, "Marriage."

This institution,
perhaps one should say enterprise
out of respect for which
one says one need not change one's mind
about a thing one has believed in,
requiring public promises
of one's intention
to fulfill a private obligation . . .

Even at the most fiduciary level, purchasing big-ticket items together commits you to behaving responsibly over the long haul, or at least for the life of the loan. Credit cards, tax returns, car payments, checking accounts, and thirty-year mortgages all make more sense when you're wed and make being wed make more sense. Take Jennifer and me, for example. People who like to wager on how much they'll earn in the near future versus the value of a house they want *now* can take out an ARM or a jumbo mortgage. We have a Mutumbo. To pay it off, live in the house, enable our daughters to live here, have their own rooms, their own bathroom, walk to school in three minutes, etc., we need to keep our marriage intact. A divorce would just about bankrupt us; worse, it would impoverish our girls. Jennifer lived through a divorce as a child and I lived through one as a parent, so we both know firsthand how devastating it would be to our children. Yet while Jennifer seems to accept this down deep in her cell structure, the algorithms of my DNA's helices insist that I Fuck Other Women. It's not really *me* feeling this, it's my helices, mind you. But since I wouldn't want my daughters' husbands' helices to get away with recommending the awful things mine do, cosmic justice dictates that Bad Jim go into retirement. Good Jim wants to stay married to Jennifer, to raise our daughters with her, to let them grow up without psychiatrists and antidepressants and custody battles, to see them off to college together, and eventually to help them raise their own sets of kids.

At my age, though, that isn't likely. It was only two or three years ago that Bea and Grace exited the diaper stage, and the joke around our house is, it won't be that long before it's Daddy's turn again—incentive enough to behave myself. As Jennifer every so often reminds me, "Till death, or Depends, do us part."

In the meantime, Goody Two-Shoes will struggle on occasion with the requisites of marriage and fatherhood. Last fall, for example, on Dads Day at Grace's preschool, Jennifer was forced to do the honors. After summarizing the curriculum, the teacher asked each student to say in whose lap she was sitting, what his job was, and so on. Eventually Grace was asked where her dad was. In her usual drama-queen fashion, she folded her arms across her chest, unfolded them, put her hands on her hips, got slightly red in the face, and huffed, "He's playing poker. He's *always* playing poker!"

Not true! As a matter of fact, I was off that day respectably supporting Grace and the rest of us by making a hoity-toity presentation at Yale University. No less an eminence than Steven Smith, the Alfred Coles Professor of Government, had invited me to talk about literature at a Master's Tea at Branford College—the literature of *poker*, but still. That eighty people crowded into the Branford reception room was due not at all to my eloquence, anticipated or actual, but to the dozen-plus hold'em games in full swing throughout Yale. I should also admit that I'd asked Professor Smith to schedule my Tea to sync up with the World Poker Finals taking place at Foxwoods, about a hundred miles northeast of New Haven. Cranking *Love and Theft* and *World Without Tears* but without really pushing my rented yellow Mustang convertible—top down, heat up, stocking cap on—I made the trip in ninety minutes, plunked down my Tea honorarium in a feeder tournament, and five hours later had a $10,200 seat in the championship event. In this sense, I guess, Grace was right.

As far as poker trips to Vegas are concerned, Grace's mom has a small problem with the concept of What Happens Here, Stays Here, especially after the city's mayor, Oscar Goodman, explained the concept: "The new brand we're creating is one of freedom based on sensuality." He's also floated the idea that legal bordellos "be used as a redevelopment tool" for downtown by turning a stretch of Fremont Street into "a little Amsterdam." Bad Jim, who travels the poker circuit alone, finds the mayor's brand of urban renewal a stroke of pure genius, whereas Jennifer's take blasphemously paraphrases that of Marge Simpson: "Homer! If I'd known there were loose women in Las Vegas, I would never have let you go!"

Which is fine. The less time I may have with Beatrice and Grace down the road, the more I need to be home with them now. Ditto for Bridget and Jennifer. When I'm not off somewhere playing poker, I can toast bears at tea parties, play catch, help the girls learn to read, even sip coffee or cocktails with their mom while attending full-dress reenactments of *Cinderella*, and maybe make love to her afterward.

As far as having another child is concerned, Jennifer feels that if a guarantee of a healthy baby were somehow obtainable, maybe we'd give it a shot. Otherwise, we're perfectly happy with Beatrice, Grace, and Bridget. We therefore need to decide how to avoid getting pregnant a little while longer. Condoms schmon-doms, we say. Ditto for coitus interruptus, a diaphragm and foam, thermometers oral or anal, or marking the calendar with x's or little red hearts. Which leaves us with tubal ligation, the Pill, a vasectomy, or abstention.

No question, it's my turn to be inconvenienced. To feel a lit-tle twinge, if need be. Jennifer has already been cut open twice for exploratory surgeries and undergone two nasty C-sections, whereas a clipjob would leave me with a scarcely discernible scar. Plus, when our daughters get married, both of us hope that their husbands will share equally in the contraceptive burden. And yet, and yet . . .

Aside from my fears about "1 percent potency," as I stupidly think of it, the best stalling argument I've mustered is that Jen-nifer won't be fertile much longer, and surely these milder Lo/Ovrals won't hurt her, especially now that she's borne and nursed our two children, especially if her doctor agrees . . .

That's Fuckwad talking, of course.

Jennifer won't get pushy about it, but we both know her deli-cate, timed-release wiles are how we ended up with our daugh-ters, not to mention my sanity, such as it is. In the meantime I'll just have to don a few more of these kiwi-flavored spring-action Rough Riders.

The truth is, us twenty-first-century studs are wan pastel pansies when it comes to our threshold for pain. Take the postmedieval experience of Samuel Pepys, the great English diarist and naval administrator, who had a vasectomy of sorts in 1658. Specifically, he underwent surgery to remove a bladder stone. Because the operation took place before 1846, the patient submitted to it without effective anesthesia, and it was rightly called "a hideously unpleasant procedure and a gamble besides." Once the scrotum was shaved, the patient was bound to a special table fitted with up-facing pegs; five brawny lads—not Jodie, not Jessica—then moved in to hold him in place even tighter. "Only five?" we might ask, since the next step called for the surgeon to insert a thin silver itinerarium through the length of the penis, this to help reposition the stone for swifter removal. And that was a walk in the *park*. As the lads flexed and grunted, the surgeon lubricated the scalpel with the milk of almonds before making *did I mention there was no anesthesia?* a three-inch incision between the anus and the scrotum. No need to worry if the patient went into convulsions, because oil of earthworms would be administered stat while the lads clutched more fiercely. The surgeon reached into the bladder with pincers and, with any luck, plucked out the stone. But instead of stitching the wound closed, he realigned the flaps of skin, smeared on a poultice of egg yolk and rose vinegar, and instructed the patient to lie still in bed for five weeks. *Very* still. (How they managed trips to the bathroom is beyond my postmodern powers of imagination.) Many patients died in the meantime, of course, but Pepys, whose stone was the size of a tennis ball, came through the ordeal with colors flying, with a single, if crucial, exception: the surgeon had accidentally severed his vasa deferentia, leaving him sterile but not, thank God and Oliver Cromwell, impotent. In effect, the happily married administrator and indefatigable ladies' man had received one of the first, if inadvertent, vasectomies.

What I'd undergo is accurately called a friendlier vasectomy.

After injecting a local and reviving me with smelling salts, the urologist would make a half-inch incision where my dick meets my scrotum. Assuming the local proved sufficiently general, he would then pull out my vasa deferentia and apply a pair of VasClips—barrettes about the size of a grain of rice—to clamp off the flow of sperm. Infinitely less painful than Pepys's procedure, VasClip-jobs also result in fewer complications than even last year's snip-and-sizzle. They're also more apt to be reversible, a noteworthy bonus when one in twenty men changes his mind down the road. The whole thing takes ten or twelve minutes in the urologist's office. Within weeks your sperm count dwindles to zero and you're back in the saddle again.

As Jennifer and I decide what to do, here's a lack-of-progress report for my fifty-second birthday, March 22, 2003: I still haven't gone in for the follow-up tests ordered by Hensrud and Gau. Why not? Because I haven't stopped drinking or significantly curtailed my eating problem and I don't wanna read the hard numbers, let alone have Martin or Hensrud or Gau see them and start chewing me out. I do drink less vodka and slightly less wine, but I'm still smoking five or ten cigarettes a month. My century-class mastery of the procrastinator's art includes excuses like: I've gone back to teaching full-time after two years off, and everyone where I work smokes. Writing the Mayo article while revising *Positively Fifth Street* left me too frazzled to go on a diet. Now that the poker book is coming out, there's *just so much to do* . . .

Eating and drinking pattern of typical day: steely resolve as I get out of bed carries me through Spartan breakfast and lunch; around 7 p.m., two or three helpings of Jennifer's cooking washed down by a couple of glasses of wine, followed by oatmeal cookies and/or the rest of the bottle till bedtime.

On the plus side, I did get the first flu shot of my life last October, following the Mayo's recommendation, and it's made a huge difference. I normally have had a couple of bouts with flu by my birthday, but this winter I didn't get sick for one day— until I flew to New York in late February to record the audio version of *Fifth Street*. As the plane descended into LaGuardia, the mucus in my sinuses, subjected to the fluctuating pressure in the fuselage, triggered mind-bending pain. Stuff like that doesn't faze cowboys like me, but I did have to spend the next two days sniffling and clearing my throat into a hypersensitive microphone. Flu shots do not cover colds.

In the meantime, Beatrice underwent a successful adenoidectomy to help her breath easier at night, and her mom finally got over a one-two punch of sinus infections. Antibiotics killed the first one, we thought, but it roared back three times as fierce a week later. This time Dr. Martin put Jennifer on Cipro, which cured the sinusitis and made her temporarily safe from an anthrax attack as Operation Iraqi Freedom got under way.

As the girls and I fend for ourselves anthraxwise, my bad habits are starting to eat me alive, both physically and mentally. In December 2003, I played in the Bellagio's Five Diamonds poker tournament. After studying T. J. Cloutier's primer *Championship Omaha* on the plane ride out, I finished fifth in the potlimit Omaha event, the first one I'd entered; T.J. himself finished first, thereby clinching the title of 2003 Player of the Year. Three years before that, after studying his primer on no-limit hold'em, I'd finished fifth in the World Series championship, the first poker tournament I'd ever played in my life; T.J. himself finished second. (This minor miracle is the basis of *Fifth Street*.) But why—and this is the thing that is killing me—why hasn't the same learning curve applied as I read Don Hensrud's *Mayo Clinic on Healthy Weight* or recall what Gerald Gau and *The Mayo Clinic Heart Book* have to say about smoking and eating, given how much is at stake?

THE SOVERAIGNE WEEDE, POUNDED SMALL

Use to get sick of seein' de weed. Use to wuk fum sun to sun in dat old terbaccy field. Wuk till my back felt lak it ready to pop in two. Marse ain' raise nothin' but terbaccy, ceptin' a little wheat an' corn for eatin', an' us black people had to look arter dat 'baccy lak it was gold.

—HENRIETTA PERRY, former slave

What are you going to do, charge me with smoking?

—SHARON STONE, *Basic Instinct*

Huron myth has it that when the land was barren, the Great Spirit Manitou sent forth a beautiful naked virgin to save her starving people. As she loped through the countryside, wherever the young woman's right hand grazed the soil, potatoes would grow in abundance; where her left hand touched, a profusion of maize would appear. Only after the world had been fertilized and the Hurons provided for did she sit down to rest. When she stood up again, on the warm patch her loins had just graced, tobacco emerged from the earth. Obsession explained. Slaves to her virginal afterglow, we're dragging and gasping our lives away seven millennia later.

The dark, bitter herb began to be cultivated in the Peruvian Andes around 5,000 B.C. The plant had a long fibrous root, erect stem, and tubular flowers: five bright yellow petals with a trumpetlike mouth. The leaves were pale green ovals, viscous and hairy, with an acrid taste and narcotic aroma. Fighting or fleeing a brushfire, someone had inhaled the smoke accidentally, liked how it smelled, waded back in to investigate, figured out how to replant it.

As B.C. became A.D. in the tobacco-free Old World, *uppowac* was both sacred and commonplace in the Aztec capital of Tenochtitlán (Mexico City), as well as among the Olmecs, Toltecs, Mayans, and Zapotecs. Within a few hundred years, the dried leaves were used throughout the Americas—in religious ritual and public ceremony, to launch wars and ratify peace treaties, to dress wounds and soothe toothache, as an enema to relieve constipation, and for pure smoking or snuffing pleasure. On a tenth-century pottery vessel unearthed at Uaxactun in Guatemala, a Mayan is depicted smoking a roll of *uppowac* leaves tied together with string. Such leaves were offered in October 1492 by the Arawaks of San Salvador as gifts to Columbus and his men. A few of them carried the leaves back to Madrid, triggering a craze for both snuff and cigars that spread throughout Europe. The Mayan verb *sik'ar*, "to smoke," became *cigar* and, eventually, *cigarette*.

By 1534, Spanish colonists were cultivating the plant on Santo Domingo and Cuba, the island whose name derived from the Taino Indian word for tobacco leaf. Traders and diplomats such as the French ambassador to Portugal, Jean Nicot de Villemain (for whom nicotine is named), touted both its pleasures and usefulness as a panacea. Nicot personally delivered Caribbean snuff to his queen, Catherine de Medici, promising that it would assuage her migraine headaches. When it did, she decreed the coarse green-gray powder Herba Regina. Doctors were soon listing thirty-five other maladies curable by smoking or sniffing tobacco.

Sir John Hawkins and his crew brought small amounts of it back to England from North America in 1565. Twenty years later, Sir Francis Drake was importing both tobacco and potatoes to England and Ireland. Londoners shunned potatoes as poisonous but had faith that tobacco cured headache, toothache, falling fingernails, worms, halitosis, lockjaw, and cancer. The Irish were partial to both.

Not everyone fell for the tobaccophiles' malarkey. As a forerunner to C. Everett Koop, Pope Urban VIII vowed to excommunicate any Catholic who smoked or used snuff in a holy place. Long before that, one of Columbus's sailors, Rodrigo de Jerez, was imprisoned by the Inquisition for "consorting with the devil" by emitting smoke from his nose and mouth. Russian czar Alexis Romanov, Ottoman sultan Murad IV, Persian shah Abbas I, and Ming emperor Chong Zhen all put to death any smoker they caught in the act.

In Elizabeth's England things played out differently. In a series of tipping points, tastemakers such as Drake, Hawkins, and Walter Raleigh began smoking the stuff in long-stemmed clay pipes. The habit was fashionable but costly, so few nonaristocrats could indulge early on. Raleigh helped change that. Handsome and eloquent, he'd suppressed an Irish rebellion at Munster and helped defeat the Spanish Armada, becoming a favorite of Queen

Elizabeth. He sent dangerously flirtatious verses her way, and once laid his cloak over a muddy puddle to keep even her petticoats virginal. Whether or not the Virgin Queen was in love with him, as many suspected, she knighted him in 1585, and his lofty status at court helped him make the case for tobacco. Pronouncing the cured Spanish leaf "divine," he advised that English colonists should grow it in Virginia. He quoted a report by Thomas Harriot, the man he'd hired to encourage colonial investment, that tobacco was excellent for "purging superfluous phlegm and other gross humours," and for opening "all the pores and passages of the nose." Harriot's report continued: "We have found many rare and wonderful proofs of the uppowac's virtues, which would themselves require a volume to relate. There is sufficient evidence in the fact that it is used by so many men and women of great calling, as well as by some learned physicians."

It would take nearly four hundred years for the medical community to decisively alter its message. In the meantime, learned physicians and others of excellent calling promoted tobacco by stratagems myriad. Raleigh's financial support of the poet Edmund Spenser, for example, seems to have yielded a Super Bowl–caliber product placement in *The Faerie Queene*, Spenser's epic allegory of the life of Elizabeth. In Book III, Canto V, after handsome Timias is grievously wounded in battle, the fair Belphoebe springs into action:

> *Into the woods thenceforth in hast she went,*
> *To seek for hearbes, that mote him remedy;*
> *For she of hearbes had great intendment,*
> *Taught of the Nymphe, which from her infancy*
> *Her noursed had in trew Nobility:*

There, whether it divine Tobacco were,
Or Panachaea, or Polygony,
She found, and brought it to her patient deare,
Who all this while lay bleeding out his hart-bloud neare.

The soveraigne weede betwixt two marbles plaine
She pounded small, and did in peeces bruze,
And then atweene her lilly handes twaine,
Into his wound the iuyce thereof did scruze,
And round about, as she could well it uze,
The flesh therewith she suppled and did steepe,
T'abate all spasme, and soke the swelling bruze,
After having searcht the intuse deepe,
She with scarfe did bind the wound fro cold to keepe.

Put *that* in your pipe and smoke it, Gerald Gau and Surgiens General! Because needless to say, Timias recovers with colors flying. He and Belphoebe live on together long and happily, sharing atweene them on their marriage bedde a crystal traye for the ash of their postcoital Marleborough Reddes. Fro cold to keepe their marriage as they reacht middle age—late twenties those days— the Nymphe taught them both to blow smoke rings, even one thro t'other, till Death did them part.

Raleigh, for his part, smote himself a grievous political wound by marrying Bess Throckmorton, a beautiful young gentlewoman of the Queen's privy chamber, but without the aging Virgin Queen's knowledge or permission. Perhaps out of jealousy, Elizabeth had them imprisoned in the Tower, where their infant son died. Things went from awful to worse when Elizabeth, too, passed away. James I, her successor, was persuaded by Robert

Cecil and others that Raleigh had plotted against his ascendancy, though James was disposed to believe it because of his hatred of the leaf Raleigh so relentlessly smoked and promoted. "There cannot be a more base, and yet hurtfull, corruption in a Countrey, then is the vile use (or other abuse) of taking tobacco in this Kingdome," wrote the king in his prescient 1604 *Counterblaste to Tobacco*. "A custome lothsome to the eye, hatefull to the Nose, harmefull to the braine, dangerous to the Lungs, and in the blacke stinking fume thereof, neerest resembling the horrible Stigian smoke of the pit that is bottomlesse."

James not only hated the smell, taste, and health hazards of tobacco but believed it was fiscally reckless to be importing so much of the stuff from the Spanish enemy. Yet when he increased the tax on tobacco by 4,000 percent, it seemed to have little effect. In 1614, as commoners took up the habit en masse, seven thousand smoke shops were open in London alone. Higher-born blokes flocked to gentlemen's clubs, where they "drank smoke" from long-stemmed clay pipes holding one twenty-fifth of an ounce, whilst their whistles and other equipment were whet by lusty meadwenches. (In *Capitalism and Material Life, 1400–1800*, Fernand Braudel reports that in 1617 executive lap dances ran three to the ha'penny, each lasting the length of one Hibernian love ballade.) Other forms of tobacco were offered by apothecaries as Medicyne.

Raleigh was convicted of treason and imprisoned once again in the Tower. His usefulness and popularity gained him reprieves over the course of thirteen years, but in 1618, James asked for his head. When Raleigh was brought to the scaffold the king, not previously known as an ironist, granted him a moment in which to smoke a last pipeful, establishing the tradition of allowing condemned prisoners a final cigarette. Bolstered by nicotine, Raleigh asked to see, up close, the ax that would slice through his neck. "This is a sharp Medicine," he declared, "but it is a Physician for all Diseases," then began to make an even pithier observation. Two *thwoks* later, onlookers noticed the lips were still moving as the head toppled off to the side. James was thoughtful enough to have it embalmed and returned in a box to Ms. Throckmorton, a tradition less widely observed.

Meanwhile, colonists at Jamestown had been trying to support themselves by manufacturing glass, pitch, tar, silk, and soap ash; by cutting timber; and by farming corn, wheat, and sassafras, as well as the native tobacco. All of these businesses failed. It wasn't until John Rolfe crossbred a sweeter strain of Trinidadian tobacco with Virginia's native leaf that things turned around for the colony. In 1612 it was agreed that Rolfe's blend "smoked pleasant, sweete and strong" and was worthy of shipment in watertight hogshead barrels to London, where connoisseurs compared it favorably with Spanish and Portuguese leaf.

The settlers also kidnapped the Indian princess Pocahontas, hoping to exchange her for colonists and weapons captured by her father, Powhatan. That exchange never occurred, but Pocahontas yielded unexpected benefits. She learned English, converted to Christianity, and fell in love with John Rolfe. Rolfe asked Powhatan for permission to marry his daughter. Hoping to mollify the colonists' lust for ever more of his territory, the Indian leader gave his blessing, and the wedding took place on April 5, 1614.

Two years later, the Jamestown Company was exporting twenty-three hundred pounds of tobacco; by 1620, almost fifty thousand pounds. (Historians have argued plausibly that one of the first Thanksgiving feasts was a celebration of the safe harvest of the 1617 tobacco crop.) The lucrative weed was now planted in every available clearing—streets, forts, cornfields, and cemeteries. Then as now, tobacco's economics were stark: it could earn growers fifty to sixty English pounds a year, while grain crops might earn them less than ten. One planter "by the meanes of six servants hath cleared at one crop a thousand pound English." The leaf was so profitable that colonists neglected to plant adequate supplies of food in its place. In the best of all possible worlds, they imagined vast new tracts of Indian territory planted with endless yellow fields of tobacco and dirt-cheap black labor to harvest it.

Perhaps the most ruinous tipping point in American history is noted in Rolfe's journal for 1619: "About the last of August came in a Dutch man of warre that sold us twenty negars." The Dutch privateer had seized Africans from a captured slave ship and sold them to the colony, which sold them to settlers as "indentured bondsmen." Market forces gathered momentum. A crash in sugar prices forced Caribbean planters to sell more and more of their slaves to the Virginians. Now that the Spanish and Portuguese monopoly of the slave trade had been broken by the Dutch, the English decided to enter the market as well. Charles II helped establish the Royal Adventures into Africa Company, authorizing in 1660 "as many ships, pinnaces, and barks as shall be thought fitting . . . for the buying, selling, bartering and exchanging of, for or with any gold, silver, negroes, slaves, goods, wares and manufactures." By 1689, the colonies were exporting more than twenty-five million pounds of tobacco. Efficiently sailing in the other direction, British slavers carried tens of thousands of men and women from Africa to the New World, the majority of them to Virginia, Maryland, and North Carolina. Despite the preference for Brazilian tobacco in other slave-trading regions, the Virginia blend was preferred in Senegambia (modern Senegal and Mali), and a vicious American circle was joined: the product of plantation slave labor was bartered for fresh waves of unlucky West Africans. Before the British slave trade was abolished on August 1, 1834, it had transported 2.6 million Africans into slavery throughout its former colonies.

Extending the circle's tangent, Virginia passed a law decreeing that "all children born in this colony shall be bond or free only according to the condition of the mother." Newly baptized slaves, in other words, could no longer sue for freedom. Slaves were prohibited from owning property, marrying, striking or testifying in court against a white person, bearing arms, or leaving their plantation without a signed pass. Punishments included whipping, branding, and execution by hanging. In 1705 the Virginia Assembly authorized lifelong slavery, and neighboring colonies quickly followed suit. "All servants imported and brought into this country, by sea or land," legislated the planters, "shall be slaves, and as such be here bought and sold notwithstanding a conversion to Christianity." *Dominus vobiscum, et cum spiritu tuo*—unless you're a negar, that is. The Solid South spoke with one voice.

Decades before we declared our independence from the crown, the first great American enterprise had been profitably established. During our war with the British, 20 percent of Virginians were slaves, and the tobacco they harvested paid the interest on war loans from France, sustained the Continental Congress, and purchased foodstuffs and muskets. Washington and Jefferson were both planters and slave owners. As Washington tried to raise funds to meet the payroll of the Continental Army, his most persistent plea was, "If you can't send money, send tobacco." The items were so interchangeable that nearly anyone could grow "cash" in his backyard—to buy food or pay off debts, taxes, or fines. Persons encouraging Negro meetings were fined a thousand pounds of tobacco, logically enough. Owners allowing their Negroes to keep horses were fined five hundred pounds. If a man wished to marry, he paid the rector of his parish in leaf, and his marriageability was measured in annual pounds of the crop.

As the war dragged along, British generals and admirals did everything they could to disrupt the tobacco trade, but the American economy was back on its feet by 1790. Foreign tobacco sales that year came to $4,355,136, a whopping 44 percent of total exports. A hundred and seventy years of tobacco cultivation had severely depleted the Chesapeake soil, however, so farmers were forced to migrate to western Virginia, then across the Appalachians through the Cumberland Gap to Kentucky. Abraham Lincoln's forebears followed this route. The grandfather he was named for was killed in Kentucky by Indians as he cleared trees from land on which he hoped to plant grain. With more and more slave-owning tobacco planters crowding west, the Lincolns and others resettled in what is now southwest Indiana in 1816, when the future president was nine. Many families moved north because of the Northwest Ordinance of 1787, which provided that no one born in the new territories north of the Ohio River should be a slave. With foodstuffs grown by white farmers to its north and slave-grown cotton and tobacco down south, the Ohio effectively became our national fault line.

By the eve of the Civil War, only half the tobacco crop, worth more than $16 million per annum by now, was being exported;

the rest was consumed by Americans. Our precious "golden leaf" had even been designed into the Corinthian columns of the Senate chambers in Washington, the room from which Jefferson Davis et al. departed south in a huff just before Lincoln was inaugurated.

To deprive the Confederacy of its richest source of war funding, the industrial North did its best to either destroy or take over the means of tobacco production. The first federal tax on tobacco was imposed in 1862, raising about $3 million in its first twelve months. The Union navy had long supplied sailors with plugs, and in 1864 the Confederate army made them part of its rations. Then as now, tobacco habits revealed class distinctions: officers preferred cigars, especially those rolled in Cuba, while infantrymen "chawed" on plugs. While it was difficult for the public to obtain either kind, soldiers helped themselves when campaigns marched them through tobacco country. Sherman's army, seduced by the sweet, "bright" tobacco of Georgia, raided stores, fields, and warehouses, killing two birds with one stone. Elsewhere, in the lulls between battles, Northern coffee was often swapped for Southern tobacco. Returning home in 1865, soldiers on both sides maintained their nicotine habits and passed them along to their brethren in every state and territory, reaching west to the Pacific. The Union had been preserved, the slaves emancipated, our national addiction established.

By the 1880s, cigarettes were widely accepted as the handiest means of consuming tobacco. Most men rolled their own, though more and more were sold ready-made in convenient little envelopes. If these packets were too flimsy, however, the product could be damaged after or, worse, before being sold. The solution was to insert a piece of cardboard, the "stiffener," to give the pack some backbone. W. Duke & Sons in Durham, North Carolina, produced four million prerolled cigarettes a day, a hundred times more than its closest competitor. The Duke company's newfangled marketing tools included printing its brand name on each pack and using collectible stiffeners—pictures of birds, flags, Civil War generals, and Base Ball players, along with educational facts. But by far the most popular stiffeners were photos of young actresses modeling risqué apparel, as Manitou might have predicted.

Cut to the twentieth century. Real men smoke, nice women don't. Marketers are going to fix that.

A female New Yorker was arrested in 1904 for smoking a cigarette in an automobile. "You can't do that on Fifth Avenue!" the constable scolded. In *Ulysses*, set in Dublin in 1904, the most scandalous development, apart from the protean language, is that the hero's wife, Molly Bloom, not only smokes Muratti's Turkish cigarettes but fantasizes about sharing one with Blazes Boylan, her appropriately monikered lover.

Per capita consumption in America in 1910 was 138 cigarettes a year. Because of their ubiquity among immigrants passing through Ellis Island, New York City accounted for a quarter of all cigarette sales. Not every New Yorker approved. A *Times* editorial praised the Non-Smokers' Protective League, saying that anything done to allay "the general and indiscriminate use of tobacco in public places, hotels, restaurants, and railroad cars, will receive the approval of everybody whose approval is worth having." The battle was joined.

During World War I, health-conscious Americans opposed to supplying the doughboys with cigarettes were accused of being traitors. Defending his nicotine addicts, General John Pershing declared: "You ask me what we need to win this war. I answer tobacco as much as bullets. Tobacco is as indispensable as the daily ration; we must have thousands of tons without delay." When the War Department duly requisitioned the entire output of Bull Durham, that company's ads trumpeted, "When our boys light up, the Huns will light out." Not to be outdone, Graham Lee Hemminger, among the profundiest poets writing in English since Spenser, illuminated the doughboys' existential predicament (and ours) with no less dazzling phosphorescence than a Hun's flare suspended by miniature parachute above the mud and barbed wire of No Man's Land:

> *Tobacco is a dirty weed,*
> *I like it.*
> *It satisfies no normal need,*
> *I like it.*
> *It makes you thin, it makes you lean,*
> *It takes the hair right off your bean.*
> *It's the worst darn stuff I've ever seen.*
> *I like it.*

Any product capable of generating that degree of customer loyalty had its advantages, especially in the Depression. Purveyors of the dirty weed continued to flourish in the late 1920s, even as most other businesses faltered. With the Huns defeated, sexuality censored by the Production Code, and alcoholic beverages prohibited by the Eighteenth Amendment, the American Tobacco Company could still hire a phalanx of leggy Manhattan debutantes to smoke Lucky Strikes while strutting down Fifth Avenue in the 1929 Easter Parade. Newspaper ads reassured nervous Nellies:

For years this has been no secret to those men who keep fit and trim. They know that Luckies *steady their nerves and do not harm their physical condition. They know that* Lucky Strike *is the favorite cigarette of many prominent athletes, who must keep in good shape. They respect the opinions of 20,679 physicians who maintain that* Luckies *are less irritating to the throat than other cigarettes. A reasonable proportion of sugar in the diet is recommended, but the authorities are overwhelming that too many fattening sweets are harmful and that too many such are eaten by the American people. So, for moderation's sake we say—"REACH FOR A* LUCKY *INSTEAD OF A SWEET."*

To further enhance their appeal among women, cigarettes were dubbed "torches of freedom." The January 8, 1932, issue of *The Harvard Alumni Bulletin* ran an ad picturing a robust coed holding ice skates and a pack of Camels. "Women," according to the ad, "because their throats are more delicate than men's, particularly appreciate relief from the hot smoke of parched dry-as-dust tobacco, and are switching to Camels everywhere."

Other marketing frontiers opened up. Female role models like Mae West, Gloria Swanson, Marlene Dietrich, and Bette Davis began inhaling seductively in popular movies. With government censors proscribing even a wet on-screen smooch, directors needed metaphorical proxies for sexual intercourse. A female character's proceptivity was indicated by her fingering a cigarette, asking for a light, inhaling smoke into her body, blowing it in a man's face. In *Now, Voyager* (1942) the neurotic spinster played by Davis blossoms into full, juicy vamphood when the dashing married guy played by Paul Henreid lights her fire. Specifically, on the moonlit balcony of their hotel, he puts two cigarettes in his mouth, lights them both, and hands one to Davis. Cut to the spinster transformed into an attractive and confident woman unrecognizable to her family and friends.

In the star-crossed sexual triangle of *Casablanca* (1942), the ritual of smoking dominates nearly every scene and visual entendre. Lauren Bacall's opening line in *To Have and Have Not* (1944) is "Anyone got a light?" Humphrey Bogart tosses her a box of matches, and the rest is romantic history. Tied up with rope in *The Big Sleep* (1946), Bogart orders Bacall to give him a cigarette, which they proceed to share in an early precursor of topping from below. Bogart's innumerable imitators all were at pains to smoke even half as seductively. Bogie too subtle for ya, Pilgrim? After the Japs have been defeated in *The Sands of Iwo Jima* (1949), John Wayne puffs out his chest and crows, "I never felt so good in my life! How about a cigarette?"

Once it became clear that a vast international audience would ape the stars' habits, film producers were offered long money to have James Bond smoke Larks in *Licence to Kill*, Lois Lane (a nonsmoker in the original comics) chain-smoke Marlboros in *Superman II*, etc., etc. Pretty soon every couple from Lucy and Ricky to Fred and Wilma to Roseanne and Dan were smoking on screens big and small. Even though it had zero interest in getting children to smoke, Philip Morris placed product in *The Muppet Movie* and *Who Framed Roger Rabbit?* Go figure. In the finale of *Grease*, Olivia Newton-John signals her metamorphosis from pony-tailed virgin to femme fatale with black spandex, heels, and a cigarette. The object of her spikier affections, John Travolta, has been smoking with unvirginal blondes ever since, though sometimes his paramour sports a dark wig, dances barefoot, and sneakily snorts his weapons-grade smack to amplify her nicotine high. The mutual crush between Scarlett Johansson and Bill Murray in *Lost in Translation* is clinched with a whispered promise we don't overhear and, before that, a half-dozen cigarettes.

From the outset, the peaks of American literature have been atmospherically clouded o'er with nicotine. Both Twain and Melville were thoroughgoing junkies, and they naturally conferred the addiction on more than a few of their characters. Stubb, named by Melville *and Freud* it would seem, uses tobacco incessantly, along with most of his fellow whalers on the *Pequod*. And who in his right mind would tell Queequeg not to smoke his tomahawk-pipe in the cheek-by-jowl bunks belowdecks? Huck Finn chaws plugs *and* smokes a pipe, unsurprising when his creator seldom appeared in public or private without cigar smoke billowing about his famous head. Twain's pal Ulysses S. Grant, one of the country's most compelling memoirists, smoked enough cigars while winning the Civil War and serving as president to give himself a fatal case of throat cancer, the very reason he failed to finish the second half of his autobiography. If he'd survived long enough to complete it, his publisher (Twain) would probably not have gone bankrupt. More recently, Carson McCullers, Saul Bellow, Cormac McCarthy, Alice Munro (a Canadian, granted, but one whose peak overshadows the forty-ninth parallel), Joyce Carol Oates, Jonathan Franzen, and Jeffrey Eugenides have all used tobacco to evoke the scarce pleasures they afford to their characters. In the so-called dirty realism of Raymond Carver, a character who smokes isn't necessarily funny or pensive or sexy; more often, he or she is doomed. Millions of us wish there were more Carver stories, but the author died at fifty of lung cancer. We also find it impossible to imagine the new Mark Twain—David Sedaris—without cigarettes.

Below literature's tree line, at an elevation where prose is often improved by the film version, we find the most famous representative of unreconstructed Confederates: big bad black-wearing Rhett Butler. Rhett's penile stogies help him preserve manly poise in defeat, or at least give him something to hide behind, while tut-tutting second fiddle Ashley Wilkes abstains from Dixie's signature bounty. Once types like these had been scorched into the popular imagination, no cigar could ever simply be a cigar.

In the face of Rhett's bluster, it took some imagination to persuade many *real* men to smoke filtered cigarettes. Enter Steve McQueen, who signaled in a Viceroy commercial that cotton tips weren't just okay for women, homosexuals, businessmen, and readers of novels. How? All the cool, slit-eyed cowboy had to do was puff brawnily away on the set of *Wanted Dead or Alive* as the scroll declared, "Thinking Man's Filter, Smoking Man's Taste."

But then came a watershed, not only for shaved heads but for manly male smokers. Yul Brynner, McQueen's costar in *The Magnificent Seven* and the king in *The King and I*, fiercely condemned smoking on *Good Morning America*. When he died a few months later of lung cancer, the American Lung Association reprised the denunciation in a commercial that opened on Brynner's tombstone, "Yul Brynner, 1920–1985," as the announcer intoned: "Ladies and gentlemen, the late Yul Brynner." Then we saw Brynner again: the sleek dome, the piercing eyes and eyebrows, the voice: "Now that I'm gone, I tell you: Don't smoke.

Whatever you do, just don't smoke." And hadn't McQueen and John Wayne died of cancer as well? Yes, they had. Suddenly, Americans had little choice but to pay grim attention as Rod Serling, who'd puffed away melodramatically in his *Twilight Zone* intros, died at fifty-one of heart disease. As Roger Maris, who'd smoked in the dugout while breaking Babe Ruth's single-season homerun record, died at fifty-one of lung cancer, reminding us that Ruth, also a smoker, had died of mouth cancer (like Freud) at fifty-three. Then there was Nat "King" Cole, forty-five, lung cancer. Bogart, fifty-seven, esophageal cancer. George Harrison, fifty-eight, lung cancer. After the *second* model for the Marlboro Man died of cancer, even the most stalwart deniers began to get the picture—too late, of course, for the hundreds of millions of us who were already dead or addicted. Peter Jennings, who'd kicked his tobacco habit for almost a decade but fell off the wagon under the pressure of reporting on September 11, 2001, died of lung cancer in August 2005.

Joe Camel, however, may have been the straw that broke the deniers' backs, at least as far as ads were concerned. With his well-hung schnozzola and dromedary charm, the cartoon spokesman (introduced in 1988 by R. J. Reynolds) shot pool and hung out at the beach with hot babes before riding a chopper to his saxophone gig at the nightclub. The dude was so cool, it wasn't long before nearly a third of American three-year-olds could match a picture of him with a cigarette, and six-year-olds associated him with the Camel brand as easily as they did Mickey with Disney. (All this according to www.media-awareness.ca.) A Joe Camel ad published in *National Lampoon* and *Rolling Stone*, whose readerships were mainly adolescent boys, included coupons for a pack of cigarettes with the purchase of another.

Reynolds even had the gumption to advise the youngest readers to "ask a kind-looking stranger to redeem it." But did the ad target children? Why, heaven forbid!

Knowing that teenage girls are obsessed with being thin, Reynolds, Philip Morris, and other companies energetically marketed smoking as a chicer alternative to dieting. Virtually every cigarette targeted at women now incorporates "thin," "slim," or "light" in its name; nearly every ad for them features a very thin model. Virginia Slims Ultra Light Menthol Superslim 120s, on sale all this week at Big Chief Cigarette Pit Stop for $29.99 a carton, may be the ultimate symptom of the Huron virgin's effluvial bequest. Hold the potatoes and corn. Light my fire.

In *Cigarettes Are Sublime*, Richard Klein makes the case that the huffiest castigations of smoking waft beyond a legitimate defense of public health to pollute what's called personal freedom. He never denies that cigarettes are bad for you but argues that especially during wartime—and when is it not?—they can be "an index of one's adult reliability." They're sublime *because* they're hazardous, he says, combining pleasure with an "intimation of mortality." *Something* is going to kill you, so it may as well be something that gives grown-ups a buzz in the meantime.

No doubt it's wiser to opt for less lethal contentments or thrills, but Klein has a point. Secondhand prudery rules in more and more jurisdictions. A smoke-free poker tournament is one thing, but now we are facing the sacrilegious prospect of a NASCAR event without cigarette sponsorship!

If it's possible to trip over yourself while riding a high horse, that's what some people are managing to do in their zeal to condemn Belphoebe's healing weede. British novelist Alexandra

Campbell solemnly promised to stop using cigarettes as a revela-
tory device in her fiction. "If Chaucer, Shakespeare and Jane
Austen could portray fully rounded characters without making
them smokers," she vowed in the *Guardian*, "then so can I."
What remains to be seen is whether she can limn them as well as
Joe Eszterhas.

Even with license to film, in Panavision and Technicolor, a
pantyless movie star uncrossing her legs, screenwriters like Eszterhas continued to exploit the smoking-equals-shagging motif. In
Basic Instinct (1992), he and director Paul Verhoeven have Sharon
Stone blow cigarette smoke in Michael Douglas's face as a come-
on, all the more titillating since she knows that, like half of the
audience, he's desperately trying to quit. To distract the kinky de-
tective (I won't call him the dick) while he tries to enter—er, in-
terrogate—her, she coolly exhales a few lungfuls and shoots him
the most notorious beaver in cinematic history. "What are you
going to do, charge me with smoking?" No, ma'am! For the film's
climax, she ties him to her bed with a long white silk scarf,
teases him in ways only a certifiable Bay Area lesbian mystery
novelist could come up with, then athletically #&¢k$ his brains
out. Will she stab him with an ice pick to trigger her sixty-ninth
orgasm? Better. Panting, exhausted, they will tenderly share a—
what else? Penises levitated, the movie grossed north of one-
twenty domestically, and a tie-in cigarette brand, Basic, was
rushed to the marketplace. The decidedly un–Jane Austenish
screenwriter henceforth could write his own ticket.

Nine years later, Eszterhas was diagnosed with throat cancer.
He'd been smoking for forty-five years, beginning at age twelve
because, as he wrote in a wrenching op-ed piece in the *Times*, "all
of my peers thought it was cool. They mostly thought it was cool

because their favorite rock and movie stars were smoking." Afraid of dying with other people's blood-flecked sputum on his hands, Eszterhas owned up to his role in that cycle: "I now find it hard to forgive myself. I have been an accomplice to the murders of untold numbers of human beings. I am admitting this only because I have made a deal with God. Spare me, I said, and I will try to stop others from committing the same crimes I did." Spare *me*, God responded, maybe because his latest self-importantly humble servant was apologizing for neither *Sliver* nor *Showgirls*, and with timing that seemed kinda fishy. Yet Eszterhas did have the grace to become a spokesman for the Cleveland Clinic's anti-smoking campaign and has probably helped save some lives. Better this Joe's conversion, I say, than the *single*-humped Joe's cartoon pandering.

I was ten or eleven when my mother's oldest brother, a divorced alcoholic sailor we called Uncle Thomas, introduced me to pinup girls, tools, Irish whiskey—for me, cut with Canada Dry—and unfiltered Luckies, the only kind sold in those days. I soon began swiping my father's Old Golds, though Luckies remained the baddest-assed brand. After dark, in the corner of our backyard, I practiced inhaling whatever smokes I could lay my hands on, so I wouldn't gag and cough when I smoked "for real" with my friends. Why did we all want to smoke for each other? For the same reasons Eszterhas mentions, as well as to impress any girl who happened by. "Jimmy, you *smoke*!? Well then I *beg* you to let me have sex with you!" Turning around as I stammer something stupid and blush, she'd purr, "If you'll just be kind enough to unsnap my bra . . ."

Ted Williams, Joe DiMaggio, and Stan Musial puffed away in

commercials for Chesterfields ("The Baseball Man's Cigarette"), but Luckies were cooler because, man, they were *toasted*, because Loose Straps Meant Flabby Tits just as certainly as Lucky Strike Meant Fine Tobacco, because the big red bull's-eye on the pack looked so hip as it beamed through the rolled-up sleeve of a T-shirt, because you couldn't be a man if you didn't smoke the same cigarettes as us, hey hey hey . . .

Yet beyond all the cultural nudges, it really came down to the chemicals. Cigarettes were the greatest things ever invented because when inhaled through the lungs, tobacco smoke— especially when doctored in the Brown & Williamson factory— imitates the action of acetylcholine, a natural neurotransmitter. What's getting transmitted is dopamine, the enzyme of pleasure, released drag by drag into our nucleus accumbens like a series of miniature orgasms. *Ah-ah-ah-ah-ah-ah-ah* . . . *aaaaaaahhh.* Mildly poisoned, the brain feels both stimulated and relaxed, zapped and spent. At first. Because after we've smoked for a while, nicotine starts to *depress* our ability to experience pleasure. As our tolerance builds, we need more and more to feel excited *or* calm. Forget about postorgasmic bliss anymore—lighting up gets reduced to mere self-medication, alleviating the withdrawal symptoms that set in when the effects of earlier doses wear off.

According to the AMA, the Royal College of Physicians, and just about every other medical group, cigarettes are as addictive as cocaine or heroin. They're cheaper because they're legal, and they trigger a less intense rush, but they insinuate themselves just as thoroughly into our cells and psychology. The FDA confirms that 84.3 percent of those who smoke a pack a day are unable to cut back. Those who make a serious effort to quit have a 95 percent failure rate. Forty percent of smokers who've had their larynx removed keep on smoking, as do almost half who've had parts of a lung taken out. Pithicize *that*, Walter Raleigh!

Some of us are more predisposed to addiction than others. Nonsmokers are twice as likely to carry a mutation in CYP2A6, the gene responsible for metabolizing nicotine. Many people carrying the more efficient version have to smoke more heavily (stronger brands and/or more total cigarettes) to compensate for the nicotine being eliminated from their system so effectively.

I don't know whether I carry that mutation, but not only was I addicted long before I got my driver's license, my grown-up job description required that I smoke, thank you very much. Every morning, before I had the temerity to write my first syllable, I had to arrange my ashtray, pack, matches, and pens *just so* above and to the right of my legal pad, all within the radius extending from my right elbow to my fingertips. Later in the day I ate snacks and drank coffee or tequila to prime my throat and brain for more smoke. And why not? Smoke helped me focus on what I'd written, the better to revise it. Every drag triggered a radiant clause or idea—at least that's the impression that emerged through the sick yellow glow emanating from this boy's mutant-reptile brain stem. The nicotine had made itself at home in my soft nervous tissue and tricked it into wanting more cigarettes. As it also began to sink into a more evolved part of my brain just how lethal they were, I grudgingly figured out ways to function while smoking less and less, though I think cutting back has cost me a couple of books. A healthy trade-off for me and my family, perhaps, but a devastating loss to World Literature!

I've now sworn off the seductive little motherfuckers 3,236 times. I've also strictly limited myself to a pack a week, two cigarettes a day, three if we go to a restaurant, and one per weekend, period. I've RSVPed to wintertime dinner parties depending on whether the hosts permitted smoking indoors. I've spent the better part of a decade smoking other people's cigarettes, on the theory that if I didn't buy my own, I would smoke less. As they got more expensive and required more chutzpah to mooch, I bought hundreds of packs for my fellow smokers, withholding a couple from each for myself: one for the road, one at my desk the next morning. Because what the hell else was I gonna do with my hands and mouth? Answer: open wide, insert food and drink, swallow, talk about quitting. Repeat.

If we Americans didn't launch the planet's tobacco craze—let's give some credit to Aztecs and Spaniards and Hurons—we certainly put it in orbit and built a few space stations and multipurpose logistics modules for it, but now we've become a leader in getting more smokers to quit. As recently as our Bicentennial, we were smoking 2,900 cigarettes per capita per year, and I personally accounted for about 7,300 of them. As a twenty-five-year-old dad both of whose grandfathers had died of smoking-related diseases and whose chain-smoking father had already had his first heart attack, I was starting to think about quitting. One reason I may have put it off was that my man Jimmy Carter promised on the campaign trail: "We're going to do all we can to make tobacco even more safe than it is now!" (Being Georgia's ex-governor apparently overcame his normal common sense and good faith.) It wasn't until 1984 that Surgeon General C. Everett Koop persuaded Congress to require that warnings be printed on cartons and packs. The antismoking cause got most of its early momentum from those ruthless little Koopian aphorisms.

Within twenty years we had chopped our annual consumption almost in half, to 1,500 per capita. For context, the Japanese have reduced theirs to 2,200, while in China consumption has risen to 1,400. (In case you emerging-markets guys are counting, that comes to more than two trillion 香烟 per annum.) In Russia it's up to a sulfurous 6,200, mostly knockoffs of American brands. In the aftermath of an aggressive antismoking campaign by the government, Scots have lowered per capita consumption to .06397 Silk Cuts per minute.

Unlike the Burmese, Americans aren't about to make cigarettes illegal, but we've collectively agreed it's a good thing to make them expensive, keep them away from children as much as possible, and protect folks from secondhand smoke. No one has any excuse for thinking they ain't lethal, but we're as free to smoke them outdoors and in nonpublic buildings as we are to eat Häagen-Dazs and sit around on our fat ass all day long. As usual, California led the way when it outlawed smoking in restaurants in 1995, in bars three years later. Unimaginable a decade ago, cool folk (identifiable these days by death-row tattoos and innominate bones "carelessly" revealed by their secondhand threads) now perch smokelessly along mahogany bars and around hold'em tables from Commerce to Mashantuckett, not to mention the Stygian pits of Olde Europe. But when even the millennium-class hedonist Kim Jong Il managed to quit, that pretty much settled it for me. On November 5, 2003, the day Grace turned four, I stopped smoking once and for all. I became overnight a fat, short, grouchy, paranoid, lactose-intolerant, infrastructure-destroying wreck, just like the Dear Leader, but a *healthier, sweeter-smelling, more kissable* fat, short, grouchy, paranoid, lactose-intolerant, infrastructure-destroying wreck. I also scaled back on the Hennessy VSOP and Plutonium Poker showdowns, though I've continued to dream of unzipping that red strip of cellophane from a fresh pack of unfiltered Luckies.

Not everyone's jumped on the Kim and Jim bandwagon, unfortunately. Film producers, for example, have been dragging their feet almost as sulkily as tobacco executives. There's plenty of artistic upside in refusing to submit to censorious prudery, so long as you don't target kids. Yet the American Lung Association reports that 61 percent of the celluloid smoking in 2004 occurred in films rated G, PG, and PG-13. Rob Reiner is among those now calling for a classification system that attaches an R to any film in which a significant character lights up. "If your movie has the F word, you get rated R," Reiner points out, "but that's a lot less harmful to a kid." Whether or not this new system flies, it's a telling inside-out variation on Hollywood's long-standing metaphor.

Much of this comes in the wake of *The Insider*, a new kind of cigarette movie. Featuring the best work of both Michael Mann and Russell Crowe (saying something in both of their cases), it dramatized the shattering experience of Jeffrey Wigand after he blew the whistle on his fellow tobacco executives. Having worked for Brown & Williamson from 1989 to 1993, Wigand offered convincing testimony on *60 Minutes* and in a deposition for a federal lawsuit against the tobacco industry: "We understood at Brown & Williamson that every cigarette we made was manipulated to make sure it delivered enough nicotine to keep smokers addicted." In case there was still any doubt.

Seven years after reaching a $246 billion settlement with the Big Five to recoup the cost of treating sick smokers, the Justice Department is pursuing another case, using a 1970 civil racketeering statute designed to prosecute gangsters. To prevail this time, the government needs to prove that tobacco companies are still acting fraudulently—likely to continue to market their products to children and play down the dangers of secondhand smoke. Wigand has testified that Brown & Williamson stopped researching safer cigarettes because one perspicacious exec worried aloud that the research "would play into the hands of an adversary" in some future lawsuit. Wigand also testified that ammonia-based additives designed to further magnify addictiveness were only kiboshed when the prototype cigarette was deemed insufficiently tasty.

The Big Five are not giving up. For every dollar the government spends on tobacco prevention, they spend twenty-three to market their products. Banned from American TV and radio, they've proven themselves eminently capable of thinking outside the box. In much the same spirit as Raleigh's poetry fellowship for Spenser, the Altria Group, parent company of Philip Morris, has offered more than $3 million in grants to visual arts groups, ranging from well-established institutions to tiny alternative spaces. Brown & Williamson, for its part, offered twenty-five Seattle artists $2,000 apiece to make art scaled to cigarette packs, in hopes that an extra degree of bohemian coolth would attach itself to Lucky Strikes. Artists boost real estate prices, after all, so why not tobacco stock?

One artist, Marianne Goldin, proposed inserting $8.50 each into two hundred packs of Luckies, effectively paying people to smoke them. B & W bought the scheme hook, line, and sinker, mailing her $2,000. But Goldin put only $1.07 into each of the packs. With the rest of the money she took her boyfriend and collaborator, Balsa, on a two-week vacation, a cunningly subversive performance she titled "Costa Rica Bienal 2004." One documentary photograph of the project shows action figures posed in an ashtray. Another shows row upon row of bright nickels, each with two pennies on top. Still another is a close-up of Balsa on a sunny stretch of beach with his back to the camera, bathing trunks lowered to the Plumber Position. And then we zero in on his buttocks, adorned with some cheerfully colorful text, one word per cheek: Lucky Strike.

NUKULAR TRANSFER

PEARLAND, TEX.—Ladies and gentlemen, Christianity offers the only viable, reasonable, definitive answer to the questions of "Where did I come from?" "Why am I here?" "Where am I going?" "Does life have any meaningful purpose?" Only Christianity offers a way to understand that physical and moral border. Only Christianity offers a comprehensive worldview that covers all areas of life and thought, every aspect of creation. Only Christianity offers a way to live in response to the realities that we find in this world. Only Christianity.

—House majority whip TOM DELAY (R-Tex.), April 2002

WASHINGTON, D.C.—Following a two-and-a-quarter-century-long trial separation, Church and State reunited in the U.S. Department of Justice pressroom on Monday. "Even through all the bad times, I knew there had to be a way to get these two old friends back together," Attorney General John Ashcroft said. "With a little counseling and faith-based intervention, I knew Church and State would work it out. It was meant to be." Effective Oct. 15, prayer will be mandatory in public school and congressional sessions will open with Holy Communion.

—*The Onion*, September 2003

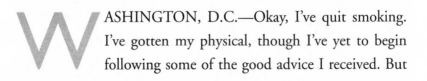ASHINGTON, D.C.—Okay, I've quit smoking. I've gotten my physical, though I've yet to begin following some of the good advice I received. But

right now I'm concentrating on a larger and longer-term health issue.

The President's Council on Bioethics has gathered in a non-descript conference room in the Wyndham Hotel, a few blocks from the White House. I'm here on assignment for *Esquire*, which is planning an issue addressing the pros and cons of the Bush administration. It's a damp, nasty Thursday, January 15, 2004, Day 1 of Week 3 of the most crucial election year since 1932, or perhaps 1860. Not to be melodramatic.

To get a better handle on the objections to embryonic stem cell research, I'm listening with as much detachment as I can muster, given my twenty-nine-year-old daughter's ongoing slow death from juvenile diabetes, one of several diseases likely to be cured by this research. (A White House fact sheet admits that "approximately 128 million Americans" are potentially affected.) Bridget has already undergone a vitrectomy—open-eye surgery to remove vision-blocking blood clots and scar tissue from her vitreous humor—and several rounds of laser treatment to help keep her retinopathy in check. During these procedures, she needs to remain awake while a gonioscope is held against her eye and an ophthalmologic surgeon burns her pigment epithelium about eighteen hundred times with two hundred milliwatts of light. In each eye. Victims of juvenile diabetes can go blind because their fluctuating blood-sugar levels cause capillaries throughout their bodies, especially in their eyes and extremities, to leak and proliferate in unhealthy ways. Bridget needs a cure for this yesterday.

Full disclosure: Even if my daughter weren't ill, I would cheer on this research with gusto. Because that's the kind of mick I am, brother. The council has seven members on my side, ten on the other. Each is a brilliant and well-informed ethicist, doctor, or legal scholar; nearly all have earned a prestigious M.D. or Ph.D. and sometimes, as in the case of Chairman Leon Kass, both. Today they're presenting in public ideas they've already published. Because some folks, like me, want to hear it from the horses' own mouths.

None of us want cloned babies or fetuses cultured in hatcheries, but a majority of Americans are willing to let a small number of embryonic stem cells be used in therapeutic research. Only embryonic stem cells are "pluripotent," capable of morphing into any kind of cell in the human body. These "differentiated" cells could then be programmed to replace diseased neurons, heart-muscle tissue, or insulin-producing islet cells. Genetically compatible with the patient, they would not be rejected by her immune system. Bona fide miracle cures are what we are talking about. Even before they're perfected, they'll dispense potent medicine: hope.

The debate around the five-table pentagon this morning has been framed, as it should be, in moral-philosophical terms. Minimal risk-to-benefit ratios for cutting-edge medical research is what the council is trying to calibrate. Thumbs-up or thumbs-down, live or die. Even so, the tone remains cordial. Members forgo honorifics and refer to one another as Frank, Leon, Karen, "my friend." Yet the rock-bottom question persists: Should "man in his hubris" or some supernatural entity write the ground rules for biomedical research?

The council most fully addresses the ethics of therapeutic cloning in Chapter 6 of *Human Cloning and Human Dignity*. The majority maintains, "albeit with regret," that embryonic stem cell research ought not to be pursued. "The cell synthesized by somatic cell nuclear transfer, no less than the fertilized egg, is a human organism in its germinal stage." Somewhat defensively, the majority adds: "In saying 'no' to cloning-for-biomedical-research, we are not closing the door on medical progress. [A]dvances in basic research and progress in the cure of disease, though not halted, might be slowed . . . It is possible that some might suffer in the future because research moved more slowly. We cannot suppose that the moral life comes without cost."

Alfonso Gomez-Lobo, the dapper metaphysician from Georgetown University, proclaimed half an hour ago in his lilting Chilean accent that "all of us were once a blastocyst." His point was that *no* blastocyst, cloned or otherwise, should ever be destroyed for its cells, however great the possible benefits. I wanted to say that we all were once ova as well, yet we don't hold a funeral each time a woman who's made love with a man has her period. That being evolved from amphibians doesn't keep us from deep-frying frogs' legs and washing them down with Corona. That people drink snake blood, roast puppy, deify cows, insist pork or veal is a no-no, and that millions of defenders of animal rights believe eating meat, even fish, is a crime, but we don't let them dictate to Smith & Wollensky or cut off government subsidies to the beef industry. Nor do we allow gun control advocates to mess with Smith & Wesson or Texas, not that it would do any good.

Gomez-Lobo and the rest of the majority argue that therapeutic cloning would put us on a slippery slope toward organ farms and test-tube babies. Their focus is on *somatic cell nuclear transfer*, in which the nucleus of an ovum is removed or deactivated, then replaced with the nucleus from a human cell donor. After chemicals coax the doctored egg to reproduce itself, what forms after five days is a *blastocyst*, a cluster of one hundred to two hundred cells, including the pluripotent stem cells prized by researchers. These could be used either in reproductive cloning, which almost no one favors, or in therapeutic cloning, to advance the field of regenerative medicine. About this epoch-making advance in Western medicine, Chairman Kass has written: "In leading laboratories, academic and industrial, new creators are confidently amassing their powers and quietly honing their skills, while on the street their evangelists are zealously prophesying a posthuman future." After September 11, he even conflated opposition to cloning and the war against terrorism: "the human future rests on our ability to steer a middle course, avoiding the inhuman Osama bin Ladens on the one side and the posthuman Brave New Worlders on the other." Not to be melodramatic.

Assuming these problems can somehow be reconciled in the political sphere as well as in the laboratory, how would therapeutic cloning actually cure a disease? From reading and talking to researchers, and with vast amounts of help from Brendan Vaughan, my brilliant young *Esquire* editor, I've gathered that the process goes something like this. A human egg is fertilized either by in vitro fertilization or by somatic cell nuclear transfer, or SCNT. First, in the sterilized micromanipulation room of a laboratory, the nucleus of an unfertilized egg is removed. No normal egg is ever fertilized; no embryo ever forms. No life is destroyed during the process. Without its genetic material, the egg becomes an empty incubator into which a donor cell is boinked by an ultrafine-bore glass pipette wielded by a steady-handed technician watching a cathode-ray screen on which the egg, magnified 250 times, resembles a fuzzy gray doughnut. Delicately manipulating a joystick, the technician maneuvers the pipette, which has a blunt mouth about twenty micrometers wide. When she hits the trigger, the pipette attaches to the egg like a vacuum nozzle sucking a beach ball.

Once the new cell has been transferred, an electrical or chemical agent coaxes it to begin reproducing itself. The incubator lab is kept at 79 humid degrees, and researchers sweat through their lab coats. But they have to work fast: once the DNA is removed, an egg will die within an hour or two.

At three to four days, the cluster of cells reaches what is called the compacted morula stage; after five to seven days, there are between one hundred and two hundred cells, called the blastocyst stage. (For perspective, a human body consists of about 100 quadrillion cells. A flake of skin or piece of stubble consists of billions and billions. One hundred and sixty-nine angels can dance on the head of a pin.) The blastocyst's inner cell mass is removed (thus "murdering" the blastocyst, if that's how you choose to think of it) and placed in a petri dish, where the embryonic stem cells can form a new line by reproducing themselves. Doctors would then be able to reprogram some of them as pancreatic islet cells for people with diabetes; as nerve cells for people suffering from Parkinson's, Alzheimer's, and spinal-cord injuries; as muscle cells for people with damaged hearts or arteries. And because they would be genetic replicas of a patient's own cells, the healing cells wouldn't be rejected by the patient's immune system. Researchers believe that most forms of cancer would eventually be curable, too.

Opponents object to the early stage of this process on the grounds that SCNT creates life in order to destroy it. Supporters argue that the destruction of blastocysts is morally acceptable because the resulting research has the potential to alleviate vast amounts of human suffering. Supporters gained momentum during the Clinton administration, but after George W. Bush took office, and especially after he appointed Dr. Kass to contour the debate here in Washington, the opponents of SCNT have been changing the government's policy.

In March 2003, Peggy Prichard Ross wrote in the *Tallahassee Democrat*:

> *In six months there is a good chance I'll be dead. This doesn't bother me nearly as much as having a president who wants to jail scientists and doctors who are trying to find cures for people with my disease [grade-three astrocytoma, an inoperable form of brain cancer]. I watched President Bush's 2003 State of the Union address from my hospital bed in Gainesville, Florida. During the speech, he urged Congress to ban "all human cloning." Unfortunately, "all human cloning" includes therapeutic cloning, which is one and the same with stem cell research. Bush likes to call it cloning because he knows it creates images of mutant or butchered babies, when, in fact, stem cell research (also known as somatic cell nuclear transfer, or SCNT) has nothing to do with babies or fetuses.*

She went on to charge that the president's opposition to this research is "scientifically unfounded" and "based on personal religious beliefs." Who can doubt this indictment holds water? She continued:

I take exception to the President using his religion to dictate public health policy. Policy should be based on science, not sectarian beliefs. The President describes himself as a compassionate conservative. But what is compassionate about outlawing vital research? What is conservative about using the federal government to dictate religion? I fully realize that my time is limited, and any cures discovered from stem cell research will be several years away. My concern is with the future generations. Almost 20,000 Americans per year will get the same type of brain cancer I did. They will be children and adults, men and women, black and white, Christian and Muslim. The disease is not hereditary, yet has no known environmental cause either. There is no rhyme or reason to who gets it and why. What we don't understand about the disease far outweighs what we do understand about it. How can any of this change if studying the very root cause of the disease is made illegal?

It may be too late for Ms. Ross, but as I wrote in *Esquire* in August 2004, "whether ES [embryonic stem] cell research should be a crime must be vigorously addressed during this year's campaign. Far more lives hang in the balance than on any issue Americans have debated in a very long time."

I also wrote that in the summer of 1979, Bridget was four and a half, a pink-cheeked, blond kindergartner with a respectable forehand and a new baby brother. In her upper abdomen, however, closer to the back than the front, her immune system suddenly attacked the islets of Langerhans in her pancreas, mistaking them for bovine serum albumin in cow milk protein. Within a couple of weeks, almost all of her insulin-producing cells had been obliterated. Without insulin, her body couldn't regulate the passage of nutrients into the cells, so she couldn't process food into energy. Long before we knew what was happening, her crystal blue eyes began sinking into gray sockets, ribs protruded through her flesh, and she was walking around in a daze. At a tryout to place her in the regular or advanced group of junior tennis students, she failed even to get a racket on balls she would have drilled a month earlier. In words that humiliate me even more now than they did in 1979, I criticized her from the sidelines for "doggin' it."

Her pediatrician referred us to an endocrinologist, who admitted her to Children's Memorial Hospital in Chicago. She began receiving insulin intravenously, and within a week began to look and feel normal. The only difference was that her islet cells couldn't be revived or replaced. As any macho dad would, I fainted and collapsed on the linoleum tiles as the doctor explained to us that the disease was chronic and incurable. Dozens of people came to see Bridget in the hospital, and the joke was to ask the nurses, "How's Jim doing?"

I eventually managed to learn that from now on the tip of one of my daughter's tiny fingers would have to be stabbed with a stainless-steel lancet three or four times a day, allowing a droplet of her blood to be smeared across a chem strip that measured the glucose in her bloodstream; this would determine the correct dosage of regular and timed-release insulin to be injected into her buttock or thigh. She would no longer be able to eat the same treats her classmates had packed into their Big Bird lunch boxes or served at their birthday parties. But at least Bridget was released fairly healthy from Children's, unlike plenty of other kids we saw there. At least she had come home.

A key notion for Dr. Kass is the Wisdom of Repugnance, also known as the Yuck Factor or, as I think of it, *Ew*-wisdom. "Repugnance is the emotional expression of deep wisdom," he writes, referring to such things as rape, murder, incest, Brave New World hatcheries . . . and therapeutic cloning. "Shallow are the souls that have forgotten how to shudder." But the shudder test is hardly foolproof and can lead to a slew of false positives. When the surgeon played by Paul Bettany removes a bullet from his own abdomen in *Master and Commander*, even Russell Crowe shudders. Yet surely the gruesome self-surgery is an excellent thing, not just for the ship's only doctor but, more important, for the sailors he still needs to heal. Whereas hamstringing researchers trying to cure diabetes makes me shudder with rage and disgust.

According to the editors of *Nature*, Kass's "support of human instinctive distaste as a fundamental moral measure of new developments suggests a determination to confront the research agenda not only with ethical discussion but also with irrational fears and pessimistic foreboding."

As a Jewish M.D. and University of Chicago classics professor, Kass has no trouble pronouncing words like *nuclear* or *vekhen lo' ye'aseh* (Hebrew for "such as ought not to be done"). He hardly fits the stereotype of the born-again hayseed embodied by John Ashcroft, Tom "Only Christianity" DeLay, and a goodly number of other Republican congressmen, not to mention our president. Kass is also out of step with Reform, Conservative, and even Orthodox rabbis, most of whom have championed therapeutic cloning. According to Laurie Zoloth of the Northwestern School of Medicine, "This is an area in which there is surprising unanimity in the Jewish community, because of the strong moral imperative to heal."

At the end of a long session, Dr. Kass finally frees himself up to be interviewed by me. Trim and energetic at sixty-five, scholarly without seeming fussy, he has a genial spirit to go with a thorough command of this complex material. Much as I disagree with him, I have no reason to doubt his goodwill. I begin by congratulating him for leading such nuanced and respectfully argued discussions for and against cloning-for-biomedical-research. I also tell him up front that, mainly because of my daughter, I want the research spigot open much wider than he and the president do.

"Some in the majority are opposed to all embryo research," he tells me. "I'm not one of them. Since the arguments about the ethics turn in part on the creation of embryos solely for research, some of the arguments about embryonic stem cell research carried over into that discussion. It's important to some of us that these were cloned embryos, and that once you've created them, you would not be able to hold the line against their implantation." Speaking, as always, in muscular sentences and pausing for paragraph breaks, he goes on: "It's been misrepresented that the council came out in opposition to embryonic stem cell research by a vote of ten to seven. It did not. It came out in favor of a ban on *all* cloning, including the cloning of embryos. Between you and me, I don't think that the stem cells you're going to get from cloned embryos are things that you want terribly much. I think that you want different kinds of stem cells, from what you care about, from what I care about." Pause. "Congress has set down certain kinds of rules about funding. They have not declared stem cell research illegal; they've said there should be no federal funding for research that involves the destruction of embryos. The president found a way to fund embryonic stem cell research on the existing lines, which means he has *liberalized* the research opportunities."

Liberalized? Only if we're talking about the handful of lines he let slide in 2001 while banning federally funded work on the hundreds of lines researchers will need to succeed. (Said presidential candidate John Kerry: "Bush's restrictions apply to 99.9 percent of potential stem cell lines that could be studied. If that's not a ban, we don't know what is.") So here we've arrived at the heart of the schizoid (some believe cynical) position on which Kass and his boss are in lockstep. By pointing to a token number of lines they approve of, they can claim to be both fundamentally righteous and squarely on the side of medical progress. When I suggest to Dr. Kass that his "liberalized" spin isn't altogether convincing, he tells me, "Those are the facts." But he also admits that grad students probably won't go into stem cell research as readily, and that many scientists "might still be worried that a new Congress might get stingy again, and that maybe there's a certain chilling effect on the field as a whole."

"Is it fair to say that the president appointed you to chair the council because he knew in advance you agreed with him about the proper limits of embryonic cell research? Or did he form his position after, or mainly because of, advice you have offered?"

"The truth is, I don't know the answer to that. I will say on the record that I think it's improper to reveal conversations we had or to speculate on the mind of the president. But I do think I know what brought me to their attention. It was not my views on stem cell research, about which I'd never written a word. I was interested for thirty-five years in trying to stop human cloning.

The president wanted to hear a discussion of the ethical issues, to hear how one would lay out the various arguments. I think it's fair to say that I did not tell him what I thought he should do." At this pause he gives off a whiff of discomfort, as a Jewish U. of C. classics professor joined at the ears with Tom DeLay and George Bush occasionally might. "Having been in and out of this field for thirty-five years, when the president of the United States asks you to serve, and you've cared about these things, there was just no way I could say no."

"So it's not that the president wanted a council to lend high-powered credentials to whatever position made red-state voters happy?"

"Look," he says, holding my eye, "the president is pro-life. You've got to acknowledge it." He gestures back toward his colleagues. "But no previous bioethics council had anything like this diversity. It's not fair to say you've got a council that's opposed to embryonic stem cell research. You have some people on this council who'd be distressed to see lots of embryos destroyed before there was any proof of efficacy. I myself am very hopeful that over the next decade we will learn an enormous amount from the existing lines. If these lines dry up but the research is promising, I can only imagine that this policy will have to be revisited. But for the time being, as a person who is in favor of seeing this research go forward, I think they're doing very well. The spigot is open."

Yet Dr. Kass and the president are leaning their full tag-team weight on the extra-long wrench that would seal up the ES cell spigot while pointing to some rusty water stains along the side—but no matter. I have to move along with my questions. "What about your hostility to in vitro fertilization?" I ask, referring to the fact that in 1971 he was putting his back into *that* wrench, claiming the procedure would lead to deformed infants. A million-plus normal IVF births down the road, he's been called everything from "bio-Luddite" and "false prophet of doom" to this hyper-sibilant mouthful: "a sixteenth-century sensibility to guide us through twenty-first-century conundrums." Which doesn't make the indictment less valid. (Okay, it does. But Kass was still wrong. He admits it.)

"I was an early critic of IVF," he tells me, "because I didn't know it was going to be safe for children. I had a change of heart in 1978, just when Louise Brown was born. In my third article, I endorsed the use of IVF in cases of marital infertility. It's been something of a libel to say that I've been an opponent of IVF all this time. Once you get the embryos in the laboratory, you have all kinds of new dilemmas about what to do with them, and I was aware of that problem. I thought that IVF might eventually lead to cloning, which it might. But on the question of IVF for infertility, at least if it's shown to be safe, I changed my mind."

It takes a good man to admit that. Even so, I believe Dr. Kass is dead wrong once again. If he'd had his way thirty years ago, we would never have found out how glorious IVF is; quite a few families I know wouldn't even exist. If Kass and his boss have their way this time, not only will we not discover the first round of cures for spinal-cord damage, diabetes, Alzheimer's, Parkinson's, and heart disease, we'll never know how many other cures we missed out on. The tragedy will become exponential.

In the 1980s, as Bridget's mother and I researched the possibilities for a cure, we were told by endocrinologists to supervise Bridget's diet and insulin routine as closely as possible, and to teach her to maintain it herself. This would reduce the risk of complications ten or twenty years down the road. The better her control over her blood sugar levels at each stage of her life, the healthier she'd be when a cure was discovered. It could even affect whether she'd be eligible for cutting-edge treatments along the way.

During the eight or nine years after her diagnosis, our well-behaved little girl dutifully followed her regimen of shots, diet, and exercise. She almost never asked, "How long do I have to take the shots, Dad? Do you know?" Having scrutinized every syllable of the Juvenile Diabetes Foundation literature and traveled to New York and St. Louis to interview researchers, I learned—or I chose to believe—that the disease would be conquered long before Bridget developed any serious complications. What I emphasized to her was that a cure would be found by the time she got her driver's license. "Just hold on till then," I'd say with a hug, trying to look as confident as possible, "and we'll have a ginormous double celebration."

At thirteen, Bridget was an A-minus student, a not-bad cello and piano player, and the starting shortstop for the Winnetka All-Stars, our town's traveling softball team. During the daylong tournaments on baked-clay diamonds in midwestern heat and humidity, she was usually the last one on the twenty-girl roster to run out of gas. We had to pack our Igloo with extra Gatorade and fruit and syringes, but by then we were used to that stuff. Bridget may have started sneaking the occasional Pepsi or candy bar with her teammates, but her overall health remained phenomenal. One mid-August Sunday, against the mighty Deerfield Does, she snagged a line drive just behind second base, stepped on the bag to double off that runner, then ran down the girl advancing from first, completing an unassisted triple play. She could not have seemed much less diseased.

The case in favor of therapeutic cloning is made by the council's minority. American society, they conclude in *Human Cloning and Human Dignity*, has "an obligation to heal the sick and relieve their suffering." ES cell research "could help save countless human lives and ameliorate untold human suffering." As for the ethical dilemmas, such research, "for the purposes presently contemplated, presents no special moral problems, and therefore should be endorsed with enthusiasm as a potential new means of gaining knowledge to serve humankind." The minority accords "no special moral status to the early-stage cloned embryo" because it has no capacity for consciousness in any form. Even more to the point, "the *potential* to become something (or someone) is hardly the same as *being* something (or someone) . . . A cloned embryo's potential to become a human person can be realized, if at all, only by the further human act of implanting the cloned blastocyst into the uterus of a woman. Such implantation is not a part of cloning-for-biomedical-research, whose aims and actual practice do not require it."

Finally, because of advances in SCNT, *any* human cell could become a person if it were doctored aggressively enough in a lab. "If mere potentiality to develop into a human being is enough to make something morally human, then every human cell has a special or inviolable moral status, a view that is patently absurd." We wouldn't be able to shampoo our hair or toss out a tampon without risking prosecution by the Justice Department.

As to whether SCNT would lead to cloned children or human-animal hybrids, council member Michael Sandel of Harvard writes: "Those who warn of slippery slopes, embryo farms, and the commodification of ova and zygotes are right to worry but wrong to assume that cloning-for-biomedical-research necessarily opens us to these dangers." Therapeutic cloning should therefore proceed "subject to regulations that embody the moral restraint appropriate to the mystery of the first stirrings of human life." Strict licensing criteria for labs, laws against commodifying ova and sperm, and measures to keep private firms from monopolizing access to stem lines offer the best hope for making ES cell research "a blessing for health rather than an episode in the erosion of our human sensibilities." Sandel and the rest of the minority conclude that it's "perfectly possible to treat a blastocyst as a clump of cells usable for lifesaving research, while prohibiting any such use of a later-stage embryo or fetus." We shouldn't outlaw *all* cloning, in other words, just because its therapeutic applications *could* be misused. Grey Goose and Escalades and Glock 22C's can certainly wreak havoc, but we don't ban their use altogether. Even Michael Jackson's face doesn't get plastic surgeons arrested.

The enlightened minority also includes Janet Rowley, the Blum-Riese Distinguished Service Professor at the Pritzker School of Medicine at the University of Chicago. "It is clear," Rowley states, "that there is an urgent need immediately to fund research on the actual potential of human embryonic stem cells to treat human disease." This morning, in fact, she politely declared that it was "hypocritical for the council to pretend the congressional ban wasn't inhibiting research." As for why we don't have a better idea of exactly *how* embryonic stem cells could be used to cure disease: "American scientists have been prevented from working on these very critical problems because of a ban on any federally funded research using cells from human embryos." The effect of the ban has been to limit stem cell research to for-profit ventures. Not only have private efforts proved relatively meager, says Rowley, "the results are largely hidden from the general scientific community and the benefits are likely to be available to the public on a very restricted basis, usually based on the ability to pay whatever price is asked."

To those like Dr. Kass who hope that adult stem cells might make cloning embryos unnecessary, Rowley insists it's unlikely that adult cells will prove to have the same unlimited capacity for renewal. "Our ignorance is profound; the potential for important medical advances is very great," she concludes. "Congress should lift the ban and establish a broadly constituted regulatory board NOW."

In person, Dr. Rowley is an elegant, hazel-eyed woman with undyed silver-brown hair pulled off her neck in a breezy chignon—a sturdy Katharine Hepburn in a dashing red wool suit, with a wallful of honors and diplomas.

"Dr. Kass makes the case that the council hasn't said anything to inhibit embryonic cell research," I remind her. (Okay, I goad her.) "He claims that Bush *opened* the spigot."

"Well, I would disagree. In our first report, the majority voted to have a moratorium on this research until there were better safeguards in place. Several council members were concerned that obtaining oocytes from women strictly for SCNT needed to be done under very careful scrutiny, and that sufficient means weren't in place yet. Another portion of the council felt adequate safeguards were already in place. Ten people favor the moratorium and seven say we've already spent a lot of time developing models for regulation. This was done under Clinton and was ready to be put in place, but the [2000] election, of course, nullified that." After a shrug of regret, she goes on. "There are people in the majority who believe a fertilized ovum is a human being and that, therefore, taking that single cell and doing anything with it is 'murder.' " She's alluding to the fact that such language widens the culture war whose Fort Sumter was *Roe v. Wade*. "Others of us agree that a fertilized ovum has the potential to become human, but we're willing to say that, under certain circumstances, if this *potential* human being could in fact lead us to save the lives of many *actual* human beings, then we think it's a matter of competing goods. Helping many, many individuals is justification for taking a single cell and using it to benefit living children and adults. Three quarters of the ova fertilized by conventional means never have a chance of becoming a child anyway. Now, to a purist, of course, that's immaterial. It's 'man in his hubris intervening,' not nature or God or whatever entity you want to invoke."

"And yet God never gets mentioned explicitly, at least not today."

"No," Rowley says, "they would generally cite moral and philosophical reasons." She's referring, I gather, to both Gomez-Lobo and Gilbert Meilaender, a bow-tie-and-suspenders sort of professor of Christian ethics at Valparaiso University, who'd spoken up to agree with his fellow majority member. "You're right, though: we usually don't talk about God. But in our very early conversations it was brought up that in Jewish law and Islamic law a developing embryo took forty days to become human.

Forty days is well within the time frame in which embryos are used for therapeutic research."

Once Rowley gets pulled away to give a speech across town, I think back to the human-development continuum in my high school biology textbook: sperms and eggs on the left, fetuses near the middle, newborn infant on the right. No pro-choice liberal would let researchers destroy anything recognizably human, just as no pro-life conservative (except for Christian Scientists and the occasional healing shaman scented with essence of springbok) objects to drawing blood from an infant, which effectively "murders" the blood. The points of contention fall somewhere between a blastocyst and the forty-day-old embryo of religious tradition. (Biblical literalists also should note that no passage of the Old or New Testament says or suggests that destroying an embryo, or even an early-stage fetus, is the moral equivalent of killing a human being.) Exactly where we draw the go/no-go line, and whether we make a distinction between what happens in a petri dish and what *could* happen but *doesn't* happen in a uterus, is determined by either spiritual/faith-based beliefs or rational/scientific principles. Religious conservatives tend to draw it at the point where spermatazoon first comes in contact with ovum (even though penetration is far from instantaneous and the fertilizing process can take a few days to form a zygote), religious liberals and secular humanists closer to the forty-day mark.

In a democratic society, then, who gets to draw it? Why not George Bush, for example, with the backing of this eminent council? Well, one reason is that the person officially charged with pushing the majority's agenda through Congress is the council's executive director, Dean Clancy. Not only was Mr. Clancy firmly and forever opposed to ES cell research before word one was uttered in the council's debate, he virulently opposes public schools and federal taxes, which makes him what most folks would call an unbalanced fanatic. Such appointments extend the Bush-Cheney pattern of loading any dice that get tossed down the policy table. Another mordant example is Mr. Bush's appointment in December 2002 of Dr. W. David Hager to an FDA committee on reproductive drugs. Hager not only opposes therapeutic cloning, he has refused to prescribe contraceptives to unmarried women; to women suffering from premenstrual syndrome, he prescribes prayer and Bible reading.

Constitutional footnote: Early in the Reagan administration, long before the salutary uses of embryonic stem cells were imagined, the Congressional Office of Technology Assessment found gene splicing both morally and scientifically legitimate. "Even if the rationale were expanded to include situations where knowledge threatens fundamental cultural values about the nature of man," the office determined, "control of research for such a reason probably would not be constitutionally admissible." The Founding Fathers designed the First Amendment to protect freedom of inquiry in general and scientific research in particular. Many bioethicists today draw an analogy between researchers and journalists. What happens in a lab may not be a free-speech issue per se, but it is so necessary to the discovery and publication of scientific data that research is protected by the right to free speech.

Yet another reason not to let Mr. Bush hogtie medical researchers is provided by the nonpartisan Union of Concerned Scientists—including twenty Nobel laureates—which complained in a February 2004 letter that the administration repeatedly censors reports written by its own scientists, stacks its advisory councils, and disbands those offering unwanted advice. "Other administrations have, on occasion, engaged in such practices," said the union, "but not so systematically or on so wide a front." On medical research, arms control, global warming, and the use of condoms, the UCS has reluctantly been convinced that the Bush administration has "misrepresented scientific knowledge and misled the public about the implications of its policies." Such a "cavalier attitude toward science," the union concluded, "jeopardizes the prosperity, defense, and health of our citizens."

The Bush-Kass bioethics majority includes Francis Fukuyama, who believes there is "a stable human 'essence' with which we are endowed by nature" and warns that we're stumbling into "a posthuman future, in which technology will give us the capacity gradually to alter that essence over time." Fair enough. But instead of Professor Fukuyama, cloning whiz Teruhiko Wakayama might be happy to advise rather differently. Instead of council member James Q. Wilson, the Reagan Professor of Public Policy at Pepperdine, Harvard's Edward O. Wilson could be asked to put in his two cents. In his book *Consilience*, the latter Wilson encourages us to let our highest ideals of human difference dovetail with the most advanced scientific research, and to see that "whatever is necessary to sustain life is also ultimately biological." Instead of pessimistically conservative columnist Charles Krauthammer ("What really ought to give us pause about research that harnesses the fantastic powers of primitive cells to develop into entire organs and even organisms is what monsters we will soon be capable of creating,") optimistically conservative columnist William Safire could be asked for his input. After

Nancy Reagan came out in support of ES cell research, Safire wrote in *The New York Times*:

> *Some argue that we should see if adult stem cells may someday do the regenerative trick. But "someday" doesn't help today's victims. Support is growing for federal regulation of new reproductive techniques, combined with approval of the use in medical research of some of the several hundred thousand frozen embryos that are stored in fertilization clinics and likely to be destroyed . . . If public opinion, already trending toward the rights of the afflicted, can be affected by the association of the warmly remembered Reagan name with a federal impetus to stem-cell research and rigorous cloning control, I say it's a good thing. If such regulatory legislation passed by Congress included a Reagan Biomedical Research Initiative at N.I.H., Bush should feel comfortable in signing it.*

Who might chair such an initiative? No doubt Janet Rowley would do a fine job, as would Douglas Melton, who chairs the department of cellular biology at Harvard. So, too, would Thomas Okarma, whose name makes him sound like a spacey Celtic hippie but who is actually a distinguished M.D.-Ph.D. who taught at Stanford before founding Geron, the company that funded the initial culturing of ES cell lines in 1998. Or how about the diabetes researcher Mehboob A. Hussain at the Beth Israel Medical Center, whose name and position themselves might have the side effect of mapping new common ground among Arabs, Muslims, Jews, and the rest of America? And don't rule out the eighty—count 'em—Nobel laureates who pleaded with President Bush in a 2002 open letter: "The discovery of human pluripotent stem cells is a significant milestone in medical research." Impeding such research, they wrote, "risks unnecessary delay for millions of patients who may die or endure needless suffering." Anticipating moral objections, their letter reminded the president that "many of the common human virus vaccines—such as measles, rubella, hepatitis A, rabies and poliovirus—have been produced in cells derived from a human fetus to the benefit of tens of millions of Americans. Thus precedent has been established for the use of fetal tissue that would otherwise be discarded."

Let's be frank. Once you appoint the right council, no one can doubt what its majority will "advise" you to do. At least as many folks with bring-us-to-our-knees credentials are more than happy to make the case in favor of therapeutic cloning. Most of our scrutiny, then, should focus on the person who appoints his advisors.

One thing this president and the majority of his council appointees can't seem to get their minds around is that human nature *evolves*. "Normal human" used to describe a four-feet-three-inch club-wielding cretin draped in gore-spattered fur. Humans used to be lucky to reach twenty-five before starving to death or getting eaten alive by hyenas. It used to be natural for a man, after impregnating a woman, to lope off in search of a new sperm receptacle, clubbing other men to death as he went, until—*blam!* And for a witch doctor to smear his gaping head wound with bat dung, a laughable remedy updated only a few millennia later to smearing it with the blood of the left vein of the Gorgon. From the perspective of these early humans, *we* are what a Cro-Magnon Charles Krauthammer would fearfully denounce as "a class of superhumans," or cavemen Kass and Fukuyama would hastily label "posthuman."

Gloriously factual though it may be, evolution is also, as James Watson put it, "damn cruel," mainly because genetic mutations have introduced about fifteen hundred diseases into human DNA. There wasn't very much we could do about it, either, until doctors like Rudolf Virchow (1821–1902) came along. Virchow was the German physician who finally convinced the scientific establishment that the basic units of life were self-replicating cells. Building on François Raspail's axiom *Omnis cellula e cellula*— every cell originates from another cell—Virchow overturned the conventional wisdom that it was the entire body, or one of its "vapours," that became sick. Yet Virchow's most radiant brain-child may be that "medicine is a social science, and politics is nothing but medicine on a large scale." We still fall woefully short of this ideal, but as medical scientists like Watson, Mayo, Rowley, Madame Curie, Jonas Salk, and Paul Farmer have shown, fighting back against disease is the most humane thing we can do. The most human.

Adding decades to our life expectancy by focusing on cells, these doctors and scientists have already changed human nature; if we let it, their tradition of secular miracles will continue. Farmer's great work with infectious diseases in Harvard laboratories, as well as with patients in Haiti, Cuba, and Russia— luminously narrated in Tracy Kidder's *Mountains Beyond Mountains*—not only saves thousands of lives but provides a stimulating (if somewhat intimidating) model of human decency. On a fantastically tinier scale, UCLA nanotechnologist James Gimzewski has figured out that the tiny moving parts of each cell can, with the right equipment, actually be listened to. Yeast cells sound beautiful when left to themselves, he discovered; when dipped in alcohol, however, they emit a creepy "screaming." Gimzewski and several doctors surmise that once the technique of sonocytology is fine-tuned a bit further, oncologists will be able to hear whether a human cell is malignant or not, leading to less work with scalpels, much more precise chemotherapy, and who knows what other good stuff. One of Gimzewski's students, Andrew Pelling, has just received the world's first Ph.D. in cell sonics, and it's exhilarating to wonder what Pelling and his generation will soon figure out how to do.

It was only more or less yesterday that we learned that working indoors and wearing hats and sunscreen all help our skin weather life on this planet, though internal cancers continue to eat us alive. If not cancer then heart disease, by far the most prolific killer in the affluent West. (Suicide bombers won't slaughter that many of us; we do it ourselves with a fork.) Even so, the folks who died childless in 1750 of scurvy, in 1850 of consumption, or in 1950 of polio would now get to smooch their great-grandchildren. We must also cope with dementia, melanoma, and stroke, maladies that people in earlier epochs almost never lived long enough to get nailed by. But whatever our epoch, we all have to face getting caught at the worst possible point on the curve of medical progress: the cowgirl's campfire is visible on the horizon, but *you* are accorded the honor of being the very last hombre to succumb to Syndrome X. "Remember when people had 'heart attacks'?" some lucky duck in 2050 will guffaw, bugging her eyes and clutching her chest in mock agony. "I mean, can you *imagine?*" This fortunate woman will be exactly as human as any victims of plague or hyenas, and a lot *more* human, in my view, than the cretin with the club. She'll just have a new set of problems, mortality above all the others. Even so, do we want to begrudge our offspring extended longevity, however fraught it may be? Her life span will seem fulsome to us, but will still seem to *her* the way Nabokov and Beckett imagined life in the middle of the twentieth century: as a brief crack of light between two infinities of darkness.

Speaking of infinities of darkness, adolescence is the first prolonged test for people suffering from type 1 diabetes. Physical routines readily followed by obedient ten-year-olds suddenly become a series of mouthwatering temptations to rebellion—against parents and authority in general, against the unrelenting regimens themselves. The flood of new hormones disrupting skin tone, academic performance, household peace, or interest in anything (like softball) besides members of the opposite sex also wreak havoc on a diabetic's cardiovascular system. Psychological anxiety goes thermonuclear, which sets off more fuming rebellion, especially if your parents are getting divorced. My doctors and parents tell me I can't smoke cigarettes? I'll retreble my efforts to buy them from 7-Eleven. And if my Dad can sneak cigarettes, there's no way in hell he can tell *me* not to smoke! And what harm can come from skipping my shot on Homecoming night? Or when I'm hanging with my girlfriends? . . . When Bridget's doctor informed her that her sugar control wasn't nearly as tight as it should be, she started skipping blood tests as well. Her mantra became "Why should I hassle with taking all this great care of myself if I'm gonna die young anyway? Huh, Dad?"

Feeling more and more impotent, I stepped up my visits to researchers, who by the early nineties were working on ways to

keep islet cells transplanted from pigs and cows from being rejected by humans. I studied reports, wrote letters to congressmen,
talked to more doctors. I imagined myself going blind, and found
myself volunteering to " ' "God" ' " to suffer this fate in her place.
My firstborn child, my beautiful daughter, Bridget, was being
ravaged from the inside out by a rapist who was winking and taking his time, and there really wasn't much I could do about it.

I began writing a novel about riding a bicycle from Chicago
to Alaska. Narrated in the voice of a young woman with diabetes,
it was an attempt to empathize as intimately as I could with the
disease-ridden angst my daughter faced every day. *Going to the
Sun* turned into a road trip connecting two love stories, and the
character of Penny Culligan is an amalgam of myself, my sister
Ellen, and Bridget. But Penny's diabetes is the plutonium rod—
potent, relentless, and toxic—fueling each strand of the narrative.
The ending is designed to evoke both the hope and desperation
the young woman feels as she pedals her way into adulthood.

The longer you have diabetes, the more severe its complications become. It's a hassle from day one to be sure, but after
fifteen or twenty years your kidneys begin to break down and
your retinopathy becomes more severe. Bridget's had diabetes for
twenty-six years now. She's frightened, exhausted, and angry.
She's also determined to overcome her long actuarial odds and
live something resembling a normal life.

But your health and self-esteem take vicious hits when you
have a chronic disease. Your skin can get spongy and sallow from
all the punctures; you also get to worry about whether you can
get pregnant, carry a baby to term, then survive long enough to
see your child enter kindergarten. "Why should I have to listen to
the history of your cold," Bridget sometimes wants to know, "or

how tough your meeting was? At least your freakin' pancreas works."

If a cure isn't developed in the next few years, Bridget will become more and more susceptible to heart attack or stroke, however diligently she takes care of herself. She may still go blind, and her kidneys might fail. As her circulatory system gets ravaged further, the dainty feet she used to lace into size 5½ softball spikes may need to be amputated.

WOO SUK HWANG, SUZI LEATHER, MIODRAG STOJKOVIC, LU GUANGXIU, AND THE GENEROUS, FARSIGHTED COWGIRLS

동해물과 백두산이 마르고 닳도록
하느님이 보우하사 우리 나라만세 東海물과 白頭山이 마르고 닳도록
하느님이 保佑하사 우리 나라萬歲

Tong-Hai Sea and Pakdoo Mountain, so long as they endure
May God bless Korea for endless ages to come!

—national anthem of South Korea

Yeah, Yeah Yeah, Yeah Yeah, Yeeeah!

—USHER

n the meantime, a thunderclap. On February 13, 2004, researchers in South Korea announced that they had succeeded
in cloning human embryos and extracting stem cells from

them. The team was led by Drs. Woo Suk Hwang and Shin Yong Moon, both of Seoul National University; one of their principal collaborators was Dr. Jose Cibelli of Michigan State. Their goal, Dr. Hwang stated forcefully, was not to clone human beings but to advance understanding of the causes and treatment of human disease.

Scientists and patients around the world hailed the results. A Chicago embryologist spoke for a lot of us by saying, "My reaction is, basically, wow!" Dr. Kass's reaction came even before the Koreans' paper was published in *Science*. "The age of human cloning has apparently arrived," he kvetched doomsdayishly. "Today, cloned blastocysts for research, tomorrow cloned blastocysts for babymaking. In my opinion, and that of the majority of the Council, the only way to prevent this from happening is for Congress to enact a comprehensive ban or moratorium on all human cloning." In much the same spirit, Carrie Gordon Earll of Focus on the Family branded the South Koreans' research "nothing short of cannibalism." Cardinal William Keeler, chairman of the Committee for Pro-Life Activities of the United States Conference of Catholic Bishops, pontificated that this use of cloning "is a sign of moral regress." But I'm here to tell you that *my* pro-life family, and I assume tens of millions of others, was thrilled. Said Bridget, "Damn! Finally. *Finally!*"

Dr. Hwang (rhymes with song) emphasized that his research was subjected to rigorous oversight by an ethics committee. It took place in test tubes and petri dishes; no embryo was, or could have been, implanted in a uterus. None of the sixteen women who donated 242 unfertilized ova were paid. Instead, these generous and farsighted Eastern medicine cowgirls (who choose to remain anonymous) volunteered to undergo a grueling regime of ovular simulation before allowing an average of fifteen eggs apiece to be surgically harvested from their ovarian follicles, all in the interests of science and improving human health. The project was funded entirely by the government of South Korea, where cloning a child is illegal. That government provides about $2 million a year for biomedical research, far less than North Korea spends per nuclear bomb and about a quarter of what we spend in Iraq every *hour*. Whatever the opposite of a bomb is, the South Koreans are trying to build it.

Dr. Hwang also noted that "almost half of our research team is Christian, including Dr. Moon, who is Methodist. At the lab, we have discussed why we have to do this work. We have asked ourselves: Is there any way to achieve the treatment of some incurable diseases without therapeutic cloning? The answer is: It is a scientist's responsibility to do this research because it is for a good purpose." In response to a question about his own religion, he said, "I am Buddhist, and I have no philosophical problem with cloning. And as you know, the basis of Buddhism is that life is recycled through reincarnation. In some ways, I think, therapeutic cloning restarts the circle of life."

Working out of the lyrically named Building 85, the South Koreans succeeded when no other team on the planet had managed to clone even a monkey embryo. Dr. Moon reported that "there is something special about Dr. Hwang's lab. It's something in our Korean culture. The micromanipulation that we did for the cloning, it's a very tedious job. But people from our part of the world are very patient, and that helped. Our researchers had an almost Zen-like sense of concentration; they could sit for ten hours in one spot and carefully manipulate the eggs. It was almost like a meditation." Said Hwang, "I also think, quite seriously, that our Korean finger techniques helped. Koreans eat with metal chopsticks, which are very slippery. We are trained from an early age how to manage them."

Most scientists agreed that synthesizing a new line of stem cells was the Koreans' most impressive feat of all. Dr. Cibelli, who helped on this part of the project, had been spending more time in Seoul because of the hostile environment Mr. Bush had created back home. Scientific advances have always come in bunches, but not under this president's auspices. This is as true for inventors of alternative energy sources as it is for regenerative medicine. Referring to his hamstrung American colleagues, Dr. Cibelli, back at home, predicted: "We will be sitting here with the best scientists in the world watching things on television."

Now that the stem cell genie is out of the bottle and into the petri dish (though not yet in the spine or the heart or the pancreas), we've arrived at the verge of an age of honest-to-God magic bullets trained on humankind's vicious diseases. Two weeks after the South Korean success was announced, New Jersey governor James McGreevey submitted a budget that would make his state the first to fund embryonic stem cell research. Like-minded proposals in Massachusetts, Wisconsin, and California also picked up steam.

In my state, Illinois, a proposal spearheaded by Comptroller Dan Hynes would provide roughly $1 billion, to be paid for with a 6 percent tax on face-lifts, breast augmentation, Botox injections, and other elective plastic surgery, but not on reconstructive procedures. Opposition to the "nip-and-tuck tax" is led by an unlikely coalition of conservative Christians and the American Society of Plastic Surgeons. The surgeons are afraid that some of their most lucrative procedures would be stigmatized in much the same way that alcohol, tobacco, and gas guzzlers have been by vice and luxury taxes. A devout Catholic, Hynes represents the socially activist wing of the church when he says that his faith compels him to help people suffering from incurable diseases.

In April 2004, the privately funded Harvard Stem Cell Institute opened with a mandate to fill the void left by the ban against federal money. On April 28, 206 members of the House— including thirty-six Republicans, more than a few pro-life stalwarts among them—sent the president a letter urging him to loosen restrictions on ES cell research. On June 4, the day before Ronald Reagan succumbed to Alzheimer's, a similarly bipartisan plea from fifty-eight senators landed on the president's desk.

John Kerry, the articulate Roman Catholic senator from Massachusetts, wrote a letter in 2002 urging Mr. Bush to fully fund stem cell research; the letter was signed by fifty-nine other senators, including several Republicans. As Kerry noted, "Compassionate conservatism could have meant lifesaving treatments for those suffering from Parkinson's and Alzheimer's disease; instead it appears to be using words of compassion to mask efforts to keep a campaign promise to conservatives . . . If, as he says, the president believes that stem cell research may have lifesaving potential for millions, he should give scientists the tools to explore it rather than have the government impose burdensome restrictions." With Republican Arlen Specter, Kerry cosponsored a Senate bill to support embryonic stem cell research. On the presidential campaign trail, Kerry charged Bush with putting "partisan politics above scientific and medical advancement. Whether it is global warming or stem cell research or AIDS, President Bush has appeased his party's right wing by ignoring scientific fact and slowing progress . . . Nothing illustrates this administration's antiscience attitude better than George Bush's cynical decision to limit research on embryonic stem cells. It was wrong for him to mislead America about Iraq's search for uranium in Africa and other aspects of the war. But to mislead the country about Americans' search for hope for their loved ones and for cures for diseases is unconscionable."

Mr. Bush bowed his head, prayed long and hard, didn't blink. Even a Coalition of the Willing probably couldn't persuade him to change his mind. His ally Tony Blair vigorously supports therapeutic cloning, after all, as do the members of the ScanBalt Stem Cell Research Network, with representatives from Denmark, Estonia, Finland, Iceland, Kaliningrad, Latvia, Lithuania, northern Germany, Norway, Poland, St. Petersburg, and Sweden. Old (Catholic) Europe, particularly under the current governments of Ireland, Spain, France, and Italy, is where therapeutic cloning is staunchly resisted.

South Korea is now the world leader, but much of the rest of East Asia has enthusiastically clambered aboard the train. To draw scientists and biotech funds into its two-million-square-foot Biopolis Park, Singapore (population: less than four million) is offering tax breaks, grants, and other incentives worth $1.3 billion. On a potentially much vaster scale, the Chinese government officially encourages ES cell research. China already has advanced programs in regenerative medicine, though details of their progress remain unclear to us, mainly because most Chinese scientists don't publish in English-language journals. Even so, *The Wall Street Journal* reports that scientists at the Xiangya Medical College claim to have cloned dozens of human embryos over the past two years for medical-research purposes; and American and Chinese scientists familiar with the field say there are at least three other teams in China doing embryo-cloning experiments. Lu Guangxiu, the professor who leads the Xiangya team, said modestly: "We're not that far behind [the West] anymore." Professor Lu's assertion that her team had cloned a human embryo two years before the U.S. company Advanced Cell Technology did it has yet to be independently verified, but several American scientists familiar with her work say her claims are credible. *The Straits Times* of Singapore reports that the Chinese have cloned more than thirty human embryos, which would give them an abundant supply of ES cells. Professor Guangxiu's team is funded by both the state and the revenue from her fertility clinic. Professor Yang Xiangzhong, a biotechnologist at the University of Connecticut who knows of Dr. Guangxiu's work, said: "She has embryos, money and the backing of the Chinese government." Paul Berg, a Nobel laureate in chemistry at Stanford, has made a somber prediction: "We will either condemn [the Chinese] as godless members of an evil empire, or we will say, 'Hey, wait a second, we can't be left out of this race.' " The ease with which we can imagine our president taking the former position makes Berg's either/or much more chilling.

Back on Blair's friendlier turf, regulators in 2004 issued a one-year license to the Newcastle Center for (Latin translation: *pro*) Life to use therapeutic cloning techniques to help find cures for diabetes, Alzheimer's, and other diseases. The license was issued by the Human Fertilization and Embryology Authority in London, which had spent three years debating every side of the legal, ethical, and medical aspects of the proposal. The HFEA is the government agency charged with licensing and monitoring all human embryo research conducted in the United Kingdom; its other main goal is to strike a balance between public accountability and protecting the confidentiality of egg donors, patients, and others. Chairperson Suzi Leather made clear that its guidelines are strictly enforced. "The HFEA is responsible for controlling the creation and use in research of embryos up to fourteen days. This includes research which may generate embryonic stem cells. All embryo research, whether publicly or privately funded, must be approved by the HFEA, and it is unlawful in this country for embryonic stem cells to be generated without a license from the HFEA." The slim, green-eyed Leather is also a prominent member of the all-name pantheon of Western medicine babehood, right up there with Trota, Florence Nightingale, Gerty Radnitz Cori, and Dorothy Crowfoot Hodgkin, the Egyptian-born Brit who took home the '64 Nobel in chemistry for developing the means to x-ray the three-dimensional structure of insulin, penicillin, and other vital molecules, leading to cheaper, more potent synthetics. Ms. Leather rides English, I presume, but whether she opts for a plain Cuban quirt or a braided Corinthian riding crop to go with La Perla, Victoria's Secret, or FCUK for her horseback rounds of unannounced lab visits, testimony before Parliament, and in camera tête-à-têtes with Mr. Blair himself has not been revealed to the staid London press corps, nor will it.

The Newcastle researchers may legally insert cell nuclei harvested from a patient's skin into human eggs from which the nuclei have been removed. Once the resulting embryo starts growing, it will be reprogrammed to produce islet or nerve cells. Dr. Miodrag Stojkovic, a member of the Newcastle team specializing in nuclear transfer techniques, told reporters: "This research should give valuable insight into the development of many diseases and benefit millions of patients. It isn't about cloning babies." Stojkovic's biggest fear is that "people think we're crazy scientists creating the latest Frankenstein." The forty-year-old native Serb could become the first doctor to use cells from a cloned human embryo to treat a human patient, provided that the HFEA approves the experiment. Stojkovic made his scientific bones cloning mammals at the University of Munich before coming to the U.K., having fled Yugoslavia in 1991 just before the Balkan wars broke out. Using a technique similar to Dr. Hwang's, Stojkovic plans to create embryos by injecting a patient's own DNA into an egg from which the genetic material has been removed. He then hopes to harvest stem cells and coax them to produce insulin in a patient with diabetes. "I have a clear conscience," says Stojkovic, who holds that life begins after fourteen days, when the nervous system begins to form.

Bridget and I will be nervously cheering him on and Googling his results with a vengeance. (She's never talked to me about this, but what scares *me* the most is that her disease may take its course just before the cure comes online.) Newcastle-upon-Tyne can be lovely, we hear, in the spring, though we'd count ourselves lucky to visit Dr. Stojkovic's clinic at any time of year, if he'll have us. Nor could we be happier winging our way to Seoul, Xiangya, Biopolis Park, or any of the ScanBalt bio-regions—except for maybe St. Petersburg, at least not till after the Neva breaks up around May Day, assuming we did have a choice.

And assuming we wouldn't be arrested, fined, and imprisoned for up to ten years under Section 298D (b) (2) of the Human Cloning Prohibition Act of 2003, also known as the Brownback Act. But I'm not so sure we can assume that.

MIDNIGHT IN THE GARDEN
OF GOOD AND EVIL

Southern trees bear a strange fruit.

—ABEL MEEROPOL, "Strange Fruit," as sung by Billie Holiday

They got Charles Darwin trapped out there on Highway 5.

—BOB DYLAN, "High Water"

American medicine had long been guided by men and women of serious learning, not religiously correct politicians. Yet as we crusade now against Islamist fundamentalism, we're headed down a slippery slope toward a fundamentalist ditch of our own—vaccination programs resisted, research curtailed, prophylaxis deemed sinful, abortion made lethal to women again, and God knows what else. Because when science and common sense get trumped by sectarianism, more bad things will happen than good. More and more Americans won't know the difference between science and theology, the very same confusion plaguing our enemies. If irony hadn't been killed on 9/11, I would say this was kinda ironic.

The framers of our Constitution deliberately omitted *God* from its language, assigning supreme power to "the People" themselves. Farsighted guys like Jefferson, Franklin, Thomas Paine, and James Madison prudently designed it to keep spiritual yearning separate from civic responsibility, and to insulate us from holy wars, crusades, prosecution of religious minorities or nonbelievers, as well as from oxymorons like "creation science" and such pop-eyed tautologies as "I am that I am." As precious few politicians did in the late eighteenth century, the founders understood that Enlightenment values—the primacy of science, rational ethics, and individual freedom—were all that separated us from the Dark Ages. That is, from alchemy and clerical paternalism, papal infallibility and monarchical whim, open sewers and plague, scapulars and bat dung, book burning and rampant illiteracy. They understood that willful credulity was the easiest path to destruction. *Sapere aude*, Enlightenment dudes liked to say. Dare to be wise.

The Rev. Timothy Dwight, the president of Yale from 1795 to 1817, condemned smallpox vaccinations as blasphemous interference with God's design. When Dr. Zabdiel Boylston (all-name Western medicine male) had used inoculation to thwart Boston's 1721 smallpox epidemic, a popular clergyman thundered, "For a man to infect a family in the morning with smallpox and pray to God in the evening against the disease is a blasphemy," branding inoculation "an encroachment on the prerogatives of Jehovah, whose right is to wound and smite," language that caused bombs to be thrown into the homes of Dr. Boylston and his cohorts. Blind faith in God bred those horrors.

Today, along with the public dismemberment of petty thieves, the murder or forced suicide of rape victims, and "unclean" rescue dogs prohibited by shariah law from sniffing through earthquake rubble, we have Christian Scientists letting their kids die in agony for want of a vaccine or appendectomy, and vital research impeded by a president who, because of his hunger for votes and incurious born-again mind-set, fails to fully grasp complex issues. His fixed-in-Sakrete mentality makes it hard for him to reconsider a war plan or domestic policy in the face of new facts—the hallmark of faith-based decision makers. Concerned, loyal citizens who ask him to retune our national priorities are branded "flip-floppers" or "anti-American." Indeed, the president's most common response to criticism is, "You know where I stand," as if that were necessarily a virtue.

By its very definition, faith is unbending belief in the absence of reasons to believe something. In its too-bright light, the disastrous results of a poor decision can be seen as God's way of testing your faith in him, not as cause for a rethink. Witness the president's jaw-dropping inability to recognize even the most obvious of his mistakes, or his blushworthy refusal to apologize for anything. As Robert Wright, the prescient author of *The Moral Animal* and *Nonzero: The Logic of Human Destiny*, noted in a *Time* op-ed piece in 2004: "People who take drastic action based on divine-feeling feelings, and view ensuing death and destruction with equanimity, have in recent years tended to be the problem, not the solution."

"I've prayed about this," George W. Bush likes to say, often in response to tough, complex policy questions. He stands, putatively as president of "We, the People," in front of banners proclaiming "King of Kings" and "Lord of Lords" to announce ostentatiously for the umpteenth time that he's been born again as a Christian.

From his appointment of John Ashcroft as Attorney General, the wet blanket he immediately used to smother cell research, and his numerous "faith based" initiatives, it was clear from the beginning that he meant to inject his personal religion into our civic life via the Christianization of government. But after September 11, 2001, he upped the ante precipitously.

He ignored the advice of Colin Powell and Richard Clarke and appointed General William Boykin to take charge of the hunt for Osama bin Laden. Boykin, while failing to track down bin Laden, informed Christian prayer meetings that George Bush was chosen by God to lead the global fight against Satan. "Why is this man in the White House?" Boykin wondered rhetorically. "The majority of Americans did not vote for him. He's in the White House because God put him there for a time such as this." There's no longer much doubt that the president believes this as well.

His support of the bill written by Senator Sam Brownback (R-Kansas) to outlaw both somatic cell nuclear transfer (making it punishable by up to ten years in prison and a $10 million fine) and receiving treatments developed in other countries using SCNT (punishable by up to ten years in prison and a $1 million fine) added a new wrinkle to the administration's research policy that has about it the stench of the witch doctor. Taken as a whole, it is one of the most unenlightened positions, with the most negative and far-reaching human consequences, ever taken by an American president.

On this and many other subjects, Mr. Bush wears his disdain for inconvenient facts on his sleeve. Honorary queer French Jewish Massachutanians like me are appalled by this mind-set, but even conservative WASP columnist George Will has thrown up his hands. "This administration cannot be trusted to govern if it cannot be counted on to think and, having thought, to have second thoughts." The complexity of honest information often generates mature second thoughts; faith, by its nature, does not. This, plus Karl Rove, is the main reason Mr. Bush is an effective politician but a disastrous chief executive.

Then there's Laura. As she romantically put it just before the 2004 Republican Convention, her husband "is the only president to ever authorize federal funding for embryonic stem cell research," proudly adding that "few people know" this. Karen Hughes or Leon Kass or Karl Rove or whoever helped edit the speech must have been counting on voters to fail to understand that this was like saying John Quincy Adams didn't sign the Kyoto Accord. The relevant and undisputed fact is that Mrs. Bush's husband is the only president ever to authorize federal rules *against* embryonic stem cell research.

Ignoring that inconvenient detail once again, this time in a speech she gave in the swing state of Pennsylvania, Mrs. Bush attempted to neutralize Nancy Reagan's potent support of embryonic cell research now that Mr. Reagan had disappeared into the abyss of end-stage Alzheimer's. "It really isn't fair to people who are watching a loved one suffer" to overstate the promise of stem cells, she scolded. "We don't know that stem cell research will provide cures for anything." Now, unless she and her husband have been making herculean efforts to keep up with the literature, disinterestedly poring over the vital bulletins posted every day from dozens of far-flung labs, this would be an example, I'm sorry to have to say, of First Lady 43 talking out of her ass about First Lady 40.

"I know how hard it is to lose someone to Alzheimer's disease," Mrs. Bush said in another speech. "I lost my father seven years ago, so this subject is never far from my heart . . . My father was eighty when he was diagnosed with this disease. This was a difficult time for my family, especially for my mother, who saw her husband slipping away bit by bit every day. In many ways we were blessed." Laura would never have thought to say *rich*, the more accurate word, but no matter. It makes just about the same difference in Texas and Washington, or anywhere high-end health care is available to those who can afford it. "My mother was able to care for my father at home and she had caretakers to help. But she was still the one who bore the greatest responsibility for his care." She meant, wrote the checks and supervised the help, although that didn't make her mother's hands-on *or* executive devotion one iota less genuine.

Even so, ridiculously wealthy and pathologically poor Americans are two sides of the same health coin. Our highest-end medicine is as good as it gets, but 45 million Americans have no health insurance whatever. Since Mr. Bush took office, the number has climbed by 4 million. Aside from South Africa, we're the only developed country without universal health coverage. We clearly have the ratios wrong, since we spend more than anyone on health care per capita—around $1.8 trillion in 2004, 15 percent of our gross domestic product, compared with 10 percent or less for other developed countries—yet we rank twenty-sixth among these countries in key measures like infant mortality, with double the rate of Sweden's, for example; we also have a substantially lower life expectancy than other first-world countries. Our system, in addition to being simply unfair, is radically inefficient. We spend 31 cents of every health care dollar on *paperwork*, for Pete's sake, compared with 17 cents in Canada. The Princeton economist Paul Krugman has calculated that "between two and three million Americans are employed by insurers and health care providers not to deliver health care, but to pass the buck for that care to someone else. And the result of all their exertions is to make the nation poorer and sicker." And I seem to recall that when Bill and Hillary Clinton tried to do something constructive and fair-minded about this, they were treated as viciously as any politicians in memory.

Where was I? Oh right, Mrs. Bush was speaking about Alzheimer's, coming up to the *really* hard part of her speech: "We are making progress against this disease every day. A new generation of drugs are under review, and more are in development." She paused, and a few in the audience clapped; the rest watched intently. The most promising protocol to cure this disease was being criminalized *as she spoke* by her husband. Her father had been eighty when he was diagnosed, with zero chance that stem cell research could ever make a difference for him. And would his daughter be nearly so sanguine if the family hadn't been able to afford such compassionate around-the-clock care? What if one of *her* daughters was diagnosed with a chronic and fatal disease, a disease she was told by thousands of credible sources might be cured via ES cell research? What if the cure was developed in Seoul or Newcastle or Biopolis Park, and you had to get on a plane and violate the Brownback Act to get treated? Passports might be revoked, white plastic handcuffs fastened on virginal wrists even, though the million-dollar fines wouldn't be a problem for the Bush family. They'd hug their sick child, gas up a Gulfstream G550 or Bombardier Skyjet, and draft a new flight plan. *Hasta la vista, America!* Who wouldn't? Whatever our circumstances, we'd all try to figure out ways to obtain the most effective therapy for ourselves and our loved ones. Having worked hard of late to keep out the wetbacks, ailing American citizens would now become brownbacks, migrating illegally in the other direction.

As a way to help deal with her cancer thirty years before it finally killed her, Susan Sontag wrote *Illness as Metaphor*, perhaps her best book. Only eighty-eight pages, it vividly demonstrates the punitive ways our culture responds to people who simply get sick. It begins: "Illness is the night-side of life, a more onerous citizenship. Everyone who is born holds dual citizenship, in the kingdom of the well and in the kingdom of the sick. Although we prefer to use only the good passport, sooner or later each of us is obliged, at least for a spell, to identify ourselves as citizens of that other place."

Even for the Bush family, Secret Service details might be withdrawn, at least for a spell. Documents would need to be forged, but no matter. They'd go. It's not even hard to imagine them elbowing their way to the front of the line at the clinic. "Oh yeah? Over my dead body," says Bridget. (If you find this Bush/Bridget scenario implausible, think of it as creation-science fiction.) I also have faith that Laura would readily do the hard time to prolong the life of Jenna or Barbara.

Not all conservative Christians attack science and reason while gorging profligately on their fruits—laws, markets, hospitals, laboratories, medical research, fancy weaponry, fancy drilling technology, fancy communications and energy systems, etc.—but the fanatical fringe surely has. They've been at it for three hundred years in this country, and their legions are multiplying. From Bangor to Hilo and Nome to Miami, but particularly in the

Deep South and Texas, fundamentalist bigots have strenuously—and quite often violently—opposed emancipation, racial equality, modern science, women's reproductive rights, voting rights acts, and the status and privileges of pretty much anyone not of their sect.

We may also recall that the president's first job in Washington was wooing these folks to vote for his dad in 1988. Under the tutelage of Falwell and GOP strategist Doug Wead, young George learned to "signal early and signal often" his born-again credentials. A plan was even hatched to isolate a television camera on his father while he listened to a Billy Graham sermon; in the script, the vice president "would be carefully following Graham's words, and at the right moment he would wipe away a tear." The Connecticut Yankee George H. W. Bush carried every state in the former Confederacy.

How can it be that 135 years after *The Descent of Man*, 65 percent of Americans can't quite get their minds around the scientific fact of evolution? That 45 percent subscribe to the creationist view? What besides *shazam* can we say to these folks? But surely we can't let them determine the best paths for science and medicine. Even though we still have the numbers on them, can we match their fanatical energy? Ultraconservative Christians are fighting a guerrilla war in at least forty states to remove questions about evolution from high school proficiency exams. They're demanding disclaimers that say evolution is "only a theory," muscling school boards to steer clear of textbooks that feature evolution and to adopt those that teach creationism.

In Dover, Pennsylvania, a new Monkey Trial took place over a high school textbook called *Biology*. The chair of Dover's curriculum committee is Bill Buckingham, a gentleman entirely comfortable sporting a red, white, and blue crucifix pin on his lapel at public meetings of the school board. Mr. Buckingham is upset because *Biology* is "laced with Darwinism." He wants the school district to adopt a text that "balances" "theories" of evolution with creationism. Why? "This country wasn't founded on Muslim beliefs or evolution," he "reasoned" at a board meeting. "This country was founded on Christianity, and our students should be taught as such." Even when creationists like this lose in court, teachers take the hint: Skirt the issue of evolution in class, unless you want a fight on your hands.

Could such shameless dumb-assedness have anything to do with the fact that our president says confusingly, "On the issue of evolution, the verdict is still out on how God created the earth"? Not that the president is a dyed-in-the-wool Holy Roller himself—much worse, he's a cold-blooded opportunist. Writing about cell research in *The Washington Post*, Michael Kinsley argued: "If the president is not a complete moron—and he probably is not—he is a hardened cynic, staging moral anguish he does not feel, pandering to people he cannot possibly agree with and sacrificing the future of many American citizens for short-term political advantage." But it's much worse than Kinsley alleges, I think. If we substitute "countless humans" for "many American citizens" and recognize that the administration's main goals are radical corporate welfare and ever deeper tax cuts for the extravagantly wealthy, we are talking about a policy that extends the ill health of hundreds of millions of people in order to reward a few thousand lavish contributors to the Republican ticket with money that no one can plausibly argue they need or deserve. WMD? Crimes against humanity? And then some. Complete moron? Hardened cynic? It really doesn't make that much difference.

What would Jesus do if he found himself in the White House? Probably not provide tax relief to billionaires while cutting health care options for destitute children. Probably not engage in loose talk about a "crusade." Who knows, though? During the run-up to the war in Iraq, Lynn and Dick Cheney's Christmas card quoted Benjamin Franklin—wildly out of context, but still: "And if a sparrow cannot fall to the ground without His notice, is it probable that an empire can rise without His aid?" As the painter Frederick (played by Max von Sydow) observed in *Hannah and Her Sisters*: "If Jesus came back and saw what was being said in his name, he'd never stop throwing up."

Is it simply inevitable that sectarian dogma will tip the electoral balance on every tough issue? Not really. Plenty of conservative Republicans, including Trent Lott, Orrin Hatch, Nancy Reagan, and William Safire, support therapeutic cloning. "I just cannot equate a child living in a womb," says Senator Hatch, "with moving toes and fingers and a beating heart, with an embryo about to be taken from the freezer and which will be lawfully discarded if we don't use it." But while many of us welcome whatever support we can get, Christopher Reeve recalled before he died that when Mrs. Reagan's husband was in office, "they were both vocally opposed to federal funding for AIDS research. Thousands of people died. But finally, because women and children across the country began to die, it became politically safe to advocate funding for AIDS research . . . It's very helpful that she's calling up senators and asking them to back therapeutic cloning to create more stem cell lines. But the way I see it, she's only doing it now because Ronnie doesn't recognize her. My question is: Why do these people have to wait until it hurts them personally?"

This is my question as well.

Jimmy Carter, our first born-again president and the man Ron and Nancy defeated, faithfully kept religion and policy separate, and the intelligence of his heart gets more and more plain every year. In the early 1960s, moderate Democrat John Kennedy went out of his way to avoid giving even the slightest impression that his Catholicism might override his duties as chief executive. John Kerry, another Yankee Catholic, gave every indication he would do the same thing during the 2004 presidential campaign.

The Bush family, however, seems unable to keep the realms separate. Campaigning for the presidency at O'Hare Airport in 1987, George H. W. was asked by a reporter whether he recognized the equal citizenship and patriotism of American atheists. "No," said the sitting vice president. "I don't know that atheists should be considered as citizens, nor should they be considered patriots. This is one nation under God." This from the Bush considered by born-again Christians, including his eldest son, to be too wishy-washy and secular.

Fortunately, we have plenty of models of balance and wisdom to go on. Thomas Jefferson. Elizabeth Cady Stanton. Walt Whitman. W.E.B. DuBois. Clarence Darrow. Emma Goldman. Hugo Black. Reinhold Niebuhr. Sandra Day O'Connor. Ruth Bader Ginsburg. We can look back with awe as a wartime Republican president struggled to reconcile his civic and spiritual responsibilities while thinking about the Emancipation Proclamation in 1862: "I am approached with the most opposite opinions and advice, and that by religious men, who are equally certain that they represent the divine will . . . I hope it will not be irreverent for me to say that if it is probable that God would reveal his will to others, on a point so connected with my duty, it might be supposed that he would reveal it directly to me . . . These are not, however, the days of miracles, and I suppose it will be granted that I am not to expect a direct revelation. I must study the plain, physical facts of the case, ascertain what is possible, and learn what appears to be wise and right." And he did.

OPEN-GLOBE TRAUMA

Narrative will never replace lasers, but . . .

—DAVID B. MORRIS, *Illness and Culture in the Postmodern Age*

I'm preachin' the word of God, I'm puttin' out your eyes.

—BOB DYLAN, "High Water"

ust before three in the afternoon on Friday the 13th of February, 2004, the day Dr. Hwang's thunderclap was reported, I was at my desk trying to integrate this wonderful news into my stem cell piece for *Esquire*—an article expressing my rage and anxiety about Bridget's health, particularly her eyesight—when Jennifer called to tell me that Grace's eye had been punctured by a two-pronged wire sticking out from the end of a magic wand at a children's birthday party. From my scalp to my bowels, I shuddered. At least one of my feet left the carpet, as though a prankster had tapped below my kneecap with a pink rubber mallet. Calling from our car, Jennifer's voice wavered between panic and her usual impatient efficiency. *Gracie's eye. Serious. Meet us at Lewy's office. Think she'll be okay, but . . .* We actually argued for almost a minute about who should pick up whom (we had an extra car that day because Jennifer's uncle Bob was visiting) and where to go first. In a raised voice I told her to drive immediately to the emergency room. The office of Peter Lewy, Grace and Bea's pediatrician, was only six blocks from the party, and Jennifer decided she could get Grace into a doctor's care sooner at Lewy's than if we risked whatever lines and red tape might be waiting at Evanston Hospital, three miles south of our house.

"But won't the ER be able to handle—"

"Just be ready!" she said, and hung up.

When she arrived in our driveway a few minutes later, I climbed in the back and held Grace, who stayed buckled into her car seat. She's a very tough cookie, as the youngest in the family often is, but now she was whimpering in pain, scrunched up as fetal as the seatbelt would allow. Bridget and Uncle Bob took Beatrice inside.

"Please let me look, Gracie girl. Daddy has to."

When she finally let me for a couple of seconds, I tried to force myself not to cringe. Didn't work. From what I could tell, Grace's right eye was shaped like an underinflated basketball someone had stepped on. Blood and some blue from her iris were leaking from two lacerations near the center of her cornea. It looked almost as dark as a shark's eye. Hugging her, trembling, I turned to her mother. "How did this happen, for fucking Christ's sake?"

Around our house, using words like *stupid* and *shut up* and *damn* is cause for immediate reprimand: "*Stupid* is not a nice word!" Grace attends a preschool called All Things Bright & Beautiful three mornings a week at the local Episcopalian church. Bea went there for three years, and Jennifer teaches there now.

This time Grace gave me a pass, but both of us knew Daddy was making the situation even worse by talking like that.

"They were playing with magic wands," Jennifer told me. "One of the tips fell off. These wires were sticking out." She showed me—a lawsuit right there! On top of which, the mother of another child at the party "was a half hour late picking them up, and they all started to get a little wild . . ." Daddy also understood that it would be inappropriate to ask Mommy which girl did this, especially while holding onto Gracie. But I asked, and she told me.

At Dr. Lewy's office, we were immediately brought into a darkened examining room. Jennifer laid Grace faceup on the table and began massaging her torso and arms, trying to keep her from touching the eye. I did the same from above Grace's head, where I stayed when Dr. Lewy walked in. Sport jacket, khakis, gray hair, couple of years from retirement. We like him, he likes us, but nobody makes any small talk. Grace was shivering, pawing her face, positively shrieking when we tried to tug her hand away so Lewy could examine her. His expressions and body language made it clear that though he wasn't having much luck seeing exactly what was wrong, the injury wasn't minor. Unable to get Vigamox drops into the eye—he was also afraid they might do more damage than good—he fixed a soft cloth patch over it and had a nurse get on the phone to make arrangements for Grace to be seen by Deborah Fishman, a pediatric ophthalmologist in Wilmette, maybe three miles away. When? "Right now," Lewy said, flooding us with relief and more terror.

We didn't talk much in the car. If an appointment with a specialist had been secured this expeditiously late on a Friday afternoon, the condition of Grace's eye must be dire. We did our best to make her less scared. Just one more doctor, okay? This one will make it all better . . .

Even though Jennifer reminds me that Dr. Fishman saw Grace very soon after we barged through her door, it wasn't nearly soon enough for me. I was dizzy with anger and helpless dread by this point, though I did understand that my manner could be counterproductive. Our only goal was to get Grace treated effectively, so I tried to let my wife take the lead.

By the time Dr. Fishman determined that Grace's injury "went too deep" for her to treat, we knew we were in a bad place. "The double laceration, combined with the depth of the punctures . . ." Stop it! *Please stop!* Though we both did our best not to let Grace know how terrified we were, Fishman's "too deep" remark multiplied our panic by an order of magnitude. Even Jennifer had started to lose it, and I knew that spelled doom, since she was the cool, rational half of the tag team. In the meantime, using her good eye, Grace had spotted a tin of what she called "lowly-pops" and asked Dr. Fishman if she please could have one.

"Oh, better not, sweetie," Fishman told her gently. Turning to Jennifer, she whispered, "If she needs to have surgery, she should have an empty stomach."

"Of course."

"If?"

Fishman told us she would try to get Grace in to see Peter Rabiah, a surgeon who *could* treat this injury, though Fishman wasn't sure it would be possible to reach him this late in the day. It has been my experience during thirty years as a parent that health crises occur only when the necessary doctor is out of town and/or the insurance claims office, in which referrals to specialists get approved, is closed, and from this I somehow inferred that Dr. Fishman thought *Monday morning* would be the best time to get Grace's eye taken care of. Measuring my words, I pressed her to arrange for us to see this Dr. Rabiah *this evening, right now, not some associate* as forcefully as I could, at one or two points edging past the limits of politeness. That Dr. Fishman didn't snap back at me, or cut me off sooner, I took as yet another clear signal that Grace was in danger of losing her eye. Somehow, some way, I backed off. But if I thought that attacking Dr. Fishman with my bare hands might get Grace in to see Dr. Rabiah one minute sooner, let alone *at all*, I was ready to launch myself vertically off my chair to accomplish it. Which meant Jennifer had to handle Grace, Dr. Fishman, and her husband while maintaining her own composure and trying to overcome spasms of nausea. She did it.

Not because but in spite of my breathing down her neck, Dr. Fishman called Children's Memorial Hospital, cut through the paging madness to find out where Rabiah was, actually got the guy on the phone, and arranged for him to look at Grace's eye. God knows how, but she did it.

They did it.

Two hours and forty minutes after the accident, we managed, with Deborah Fishman's and, less directly, Peter Lewy's help, to deliver Grace into the hands of Peter Rabiah, an ophthalmological surgeon at Children's, where Bridget had been admitted after her diagnosis twenty-five years earlier. (To show how much I've grown as a person since then, this time I didn't criticize my four-year-old daughter for "doggin' it" or asking for a lollipop.) Another huge factor was our Cigna insurance card, plastically

representing a policy issued for free by my employer, the Art Institute of Chicago, whose policy is handled by Fred Novy. For a
bimonthly payroll deduction of $115.60, my family is covered as
well. Once Grace's primary care physician (Lewy) set the ball
rolling, whoever saw Grace after that, and whatever procedure he
or she performed, would be covered.

It turned out that Dr. Rabiah was only up our way because of
a weekly staff meeting at Glenbrook Hospital. Normally he was
off duty by five, but the meeting ran long for some reason. His
colleagues and nurses and office staff had all gone home as he
waited for us in his suite of dark offices. Medium height and
build, pale olive skin, balding, dark hair, visibly tired at the end
of a long day and week—the most beautiful person we'd ever laid
eyes on. We introduced ourselves and thanked him profusely for
being there.

"Let me have a look."

But Grace wouldn't let him, at least not in the ways and from
all the angles he wanted to. She was simply too scared, in too
much pain, to sit still for her third doctor, especially after we'd
promised during the previous consultations that each was the last
one she'd have to submit to. She was also getting hungry and
thirsty. Even with both parents reassuring her while trying to
hold her in place, Rabiah was unable to examine her thoroughly.
There were drops he wanted to put in, a device he wanted to use.
Nothing doing. By simply covering Grace's left eye with his hand,
however, he was able to determine that she had zero vision in the
right. After looking a little while longer, cocking his head this
way and that, he told us, "She has two full-thickness corneal lacerations, one at about the twelve-o'clock position and one at
about two o'clock. The lacerations are midperipheral, and her—"

"Meaning?"

"Not directly over the visual axis, though it's close."

Bewildered and crazed, I just nodded.

"The anterior chamber is shallow," he said, "though formed. Some iris strands have prolapsed into the two lacerations, where they've become incarcerated." His soft-spoken voice made all this easier to understand but also more devastating. I could tell it was *killing* my wife. But we listened; he talked. He needed to put Grace under general anesthesia to thoroughly examine the eye and try to repair it.

Now we gaped at him, begging for promises, answers, predictions. This was a seasoned pediatric ophthalmologist, an exquisitely talented surgeon, and Grace's only hope. He was not optimistic. "This is a serious open-globe injury," he told us in a not-quite-neutral tone of voice. "The visual prognosis is guarded." As Jennifer put Grace's coat on her in the waiting area, he also had no choice but to hold my eye for a few extra beats: "You need to be aware that children this age can die under general anesthesia."

We sat with Grace on a couch as he called Evanston Hospital and reserved an OR. I didn't mutter, "Why not just operate here?" out loud, but he answered that question a few moments later.

"Evanston Hospital has a more sophisticated Trauma Center."

He in his car and we in ours, we drove the ten miles to Evanston. Using Jennifer's cell phone, I did my best to "vet" Peter Rabiah by calling Scott Rosen, an ophthalmologist I used to play tennis with. Scott assured me that Grace was in very good hands, and he volunteered to assist if Rabiah needed help. I thanked him. But wasn't Scott's glowing assessment of Rabiah transparently designed to reassure a panicked friend? And what would we have done if Scott had told me otherwise—canceled the emergency operation while we tried to link up with a more well-thought-of surgeon, someone who also happened to be on call Friday night?

I didn't tell Jennifer what Rabiah had said about anesthesia. She understood that already, didn't need to hear those foul words. We were altogether helpless in this good doctor's hands, but we knew we were lucky to be there. If Fishman had reached him ten minutes later, he would have been out the door, headed home or to a restaurant, starting his weekend with a vodka martini perhaps, effectively shunting Grace's blind eye under the knife of a junior associate.

Grace didn't believe us, of course, when we promised her that the *next* stop would be the last of the night. I wasn't that certain myself.

At Evanston, Jennifer did most of the signing and talking. She knew the story of the injury firsthand, as well as the embarrassing fact that Grace's dad couldn't bear to think about the hideous details, let alone rehearse them for every new "intake specialist" who strolled into the room. She knew that when a doctor was explaining diabetes to me after Bridget was diagnosed, I fainted and collapsed on the floor. Now I was standing here holding my third daughter, hoping I wouldn't pass out. I was frantic to get the surgery under way but impotent to make anything happen. *Not fainting* was the extent of my usefulness.

As it dawned on Grace that this might well be the last stop of her very bad day, she began to display more of her signature attitude. As each new green- or blue-gowned specialist said hello and asked the patient's name, Grace began shooting back, "I already told you! What's *your* name?" To a Thai technician who introduced herself as Sirikit, she said, "*That's* a funny name." Her feistiness embarrassed us but at least seemed to indicate that she wasn't in horrible shape overall. But what did it say about her eye?

Besides being sassy as hell, Grace is a roughhouser, one of the few girls her age who prefer boys as playmates. From now on she was gonna have to behave *much* more sedately. It was also starting to sink in that Grace was just as likely to have been the one whipping a wand around other girls' faces. Even so, I wanted to smack the little girl who had slashed her.

We were soon introduced to a confident, muscular young African American guy with a gleaming brown skull, big white teeth, and ripped ceps emerging from his short-sleeved hospital top. He wore a chain around his neck—no delicate links to display a modest crucifix or St. Christopher's medal, but a chunky inch-wide affair fitted tightly below his Adam's apple. It appeared to signify both domination and submission, probably with a sexual subtext. Was this hard, kinky brother the orderly charged with wheeling our vulnerable daughter into the operating room? No, he was Dr. Rouse, who'd be assisting Dr. Rabiah in the surgery.

The anesthesiologist was an Egyptian-looking guy who resembled Omar Sharif, only stockier. He pressed us to be precise about when Grace had eaten last. (Two-thirty p.m.) What? (Birthday cake.) How much? (Just one piece.)

At last an orderly with no chains of any sort around her neck arrived to wheel Grace through the door, beyond which Peter Rabiah was waiting.

How annihilatingly ridiculous it was for me to pray that the surgery would be successful, though I caught myself doing it, after a fashion at least. As I'd written in the stem cell piece that very afternoon: "Religion evolved to help us cope with poverty, imprisonment, fear of death, and other bad things, and that's fine. But is some white-bearded guy named Jehovah or Olodumare, God or Allah really out there? In here? On a throne up in heaven, above and to the left of Cloud 9?" But that's pretty much where I was aiming my supplications as Jennifer called home to check up on Beatrice. Nor could I help picturing Grace on the table, faceup under a microscope, eye pulled wide open *and cut,* surrounded by three dark strange men and all those damn lights and equipment. "Because once your blipping EEG line goes flat, it's going to be all she wrote."

Two hours later, Rabiah comes out to report the initial results. Neither optimism nor pessimism colors his voice. "She has a long haul ahead of her, but her retina was untouched, and her lens, while traumatized, was intact." He'd been able to inject a gel into her eye, he says, to rebuild the cornea and help it begin to repressurize. He lets one of us—Jennifer—go back to be there when Gracie comes to.

My gratitude and relief upon hearing his guardedly hopeful prognosis are so overwhelming that I don't know what to say. "It didn't look like much of an eye this afternoon."

He agrees.

"Was it worse because there were two?"

"The double punctures didn't change much in terms of her vision, because it depended where they were exactly, and neither was in the worst spot."

Two punctures doubled the opportunities for infection, how-ever. We'd have to be extra vigilant with antibacterial drops. I promised him we would be and thanked him and thanked him and thanked him.

How did he learn to do this miraculous thing? By having brains and steady hands but also by working his ass off.

Googling Peter K. Rabiah, we find that he graduated from the University of Michigan Medical School in 1988, followed by a residency in ophthalmology at the University of Illinois. Two-year fellowships in uveitis (inflammation of the pigmented layer of the eye) at Illinois and pediatric ophthalmology at UCLA. Board-certified in ophthalmology, 1994. Graduating from college around 1984 made him a little over forty, I figured; his name and features made him Arab American.

He wouldn't have been hired to work and teach at Children's Memorial, one of the best pediatric hospitals anywhere, if he wasn't really good at his job going in. After that, during ten years of practice, it's fair to assume he got better and better: sharper diagnostic skills, more precision under the microscope, more effective follow-up protocols. An accomplished healer to begin with, he got used to dealing with some of the toughest cases in Chicago, as well as the traumas and complications that ophthal-mologists throughout the Midwest couldn't handle.

Here's the kicker. Google also takes us to the Web site of the International Centre for Eye Health, where we learn that five months before Grace's accident, someone had published a paper called "Penetrating Needle Injury of the Eye Causing Cataract in Children" in the distinguished journal *Ophthalmology*. The author had studied "the presentation, management, and outcome of children with cataract caused by ocular needle penetration." In what is called a "noncomparative interventional case series," he surgically treated forty-two children with cataracts caused by needle penetration, almost exactly the injury Gracie would suffer. Endophthalmitis (infection of the intraocular cavities that can lead to decreased vision or permanent loss of vision) developed in fourteen cases. To eradicate a blind and painful eye that can result, enucleation (removal) is often required. I swallowed, read on. "With a mean postoperative follow-up of 2.3 years, the best-corrected visual acuity was 20/40 or better in 19 cases, 20/50 to 20/80 in 7, 20/100 to counting fingers in 6, light perception in 1, no light perception in 6, and undetermined in 3. Eyes with endophthalmitis and/or retinal detachment had a worse visual prognosis." The author concluded: "Ocular penetration causing cataract occurred in children during unsupervised play with inadequately stored or disposed of hypodermic or sewing needles. Endophthalmitis occurred frequently in injuries caused by hypodermic needles but not in those caused by sewing needles. Visual outcome after management was good in approximately half of the cases especially if endophthalmitis or retinal detachment did not develop." The author was Peter K. Rabiah.

The guy we'd lucked into is the very surgeon you'd want manning the microscope and supervising the aftercare if your child's eye got injured this way. If his study had been written less recently, the state of the art might have changed. As it was, Peter Rabiah was almost ridiculously well prepared to save Grace's eye. The care she received was as good as it gets, probably could not be improved on. If only we'd known this as we drove her to the hospital that night, or argued about where to go first! Thank God

Dr. Rabiah was available, we kept saying to ourselves and telling each other. God forbid that a second-rate surgeon would've handled the case . . .

What's the difference between God and a surgeon? God doesn't think he's a surgeon. A plumber attended to a leaking faucet at a surgeon's house. After a two-minute job, he demanded a hundred and fifty dollars. The surgeon exclaimed, "I don't even charge that much and I'm a surgeon!" The plumber replied, "I didn't either when I was a surgeon. That's why I switched to plumbing." Then there's the young girl who tells her parents, "A boy in my class asked me to play doctor." Oh, dear, say her parents, wringing their hands. What happened, honey? "He made me wait forty-five minutes then double-billed the insurance company." How many doctors does it take to change a lightbulb? Depends on whether it has health insurance. All doctors have excellent tans, by the way. They couldn't care less about patients, sprinting through rounds so as not to miss tee times or the most excellent wind-surfing conditions. They're arrogant bastards (and, lately, bitches) who think they have all the answers. They suck.

The blood sport of doctor bashing is all well and good and quite often terribly funny. No doubt many doctors deserve heaps of enmity and or prison time, if not Texas justice itself. Even so, a whole lot of folks underestimate how arduous and expensive it is to obtain a diploma that simply gets your foot in the door of a serious laboratory or teaching hospital. A full-scale scientific or medical education, from college through postgraduate work, costs more than a million dollars. Certainly the prospect of a handsome income is a motivating factor, but so is pure altruistic *heart*. How else could these folks make it through the long educational process? Premed types and science wonks have to skip a lot of tailgate parties, hot dates, and greet-the-dawn poker sessions to get the kind of grades that make them eligible for med school or high-powered Ph.D. programs. Once they get admitted (to med school at least), they can kiss their social and nightlife good-bye. Yet delaying gratification and working their ass off in med school barely prepares them for the staggering grind that interns put up with: fifty-hour days in a series of life-and-death situations for salaries on a par with those of nannies and construction workers, not a twelfth of what banjo-hitting utility infielders make. What nannies and laborers do is plenty important, but we owe smart M.D.'s and lab rats our lives.

When Peter Rabiah was in his mid-thirties, he was still going to school to learn how to keep children from going blind. In fact, because of the way the literature of his specialty happily keeps expanding (in part because of him), he'll be in school until he retires. Did I mention that *he keeps injured and sick children from going blind*, but that the way he carries himself in his practice couldn't be more unassuming? If a child needs his expertise late of a Friday, when he's already halfway out the door, he stays on for several more hours. (This happens irrespective of insurance coverage, by the way, because the hospital group pays him a salary that doesn't depend on how much they collect from individual patients. Plus it's virtually unimaginable that *any* doctor would send an injured but uninsured child on her way. Her family might get dunned till the cows come home, but her eye will get treated just the same.) How much does Rabiah earn? Middle six figures, I'd guess. I'd also guess that without the possibility of being well compensated, his and a lot of other excellent doctoring, not to mention breakthroughs in the laboratory, simply wouldn't happen. Whatever income and status and *tans* these people derive by keeping us out of the clinic or crematorium, or heading off enucleation, they richly deserve.

Grace spent three days in Evanston Hospital receiving IV antibiotics. Jennifer stayed in the room around the clock and slept in Grace's bed with her. During the day she took a crash course in eyedrop technique and suture care, both critical to the healing process. She must have been a pretty good student because Grace was sent home sooner than expected. Along with her perforated metal eye shield and cool plastic ID bracelet, she's packing prescriptions for Vigamox (an antibacterial to ward off endophthalmitis and other infections), atropine (synthetic belladonna to paralyze the sphincter muscle of the iris, causing dilation; also to reduce pain and prevent complications), and Pred Forte (a steroid to maintain healthy pressure and reduce inflammation). Drugs this potent, especially in combination, especially in a child's eye, need precise management. We need to get each one into the eye three or four times a day, but not at the same time. As the dosages change, the protocol gets so complicated that Jennifer devises a sticker chart to keep it all straight, peeling off Hello Kitty stickers as rewards for holding still. The first few bandage brands we use to hold the shield in place irritate Grace's pale skin; after two return trips to the drugstore, the Johnson & Johnson First Aid HURT-FREE Tape finally works. We also stock a "treasure chest" with Hello Kitty toys, Play-Doh, and jungle-cat coloring books, from which Grace can choose one item at the end of each week that she "helps Mommy help me get better." (She'll get to pick one anyway, of course, but it still often works as a carrot when she's overexcited or not in the mood for more drops.) In the meantime, she can't go to school. No jumping, running, skipping, somersaulting, ice-skating, bike riding. Can't even go to the park because dirt or sand might get tossed or blown into her eye. Washing her hair takes an hour. No play dates for the first month or so, not even between drop applications; the responsibility would simply be too much to lay on another parent. In early March, Daddy begins a paperback book tour. On April 7, with Daddy promoting his book in Las Vegas, we *move*.

Forty-six days after the accident—"Seems like forty-seven," says Mommy—Grace once again goes under general anesthesia so Rabiah can remove the stitches. This time it's outpatient surgery, though still a big deal. It goes well. Easy as pie, as a matter of fact, especially for Daddy, since he's off in L.A. signing books.

At the post-op appointment three days later, Daddy is around to notice on Rabiah's wall a framed watercolor of a yellow castle—fanciful, Chagallish, with tulips and palm trees growing from its walls, a salmon for a weathervane, a girl flying above the turrets. Grace has become kinda weepy, and we point out the picture to help her calm down.

"I miss Dr. Rabiah!" Though neither of us asks her why, she adds, "He has a Rafiki toy from *The Lion King*!"

When smiling Nurse Rebecca tries to put in drops that would illuminate any scarring in the eye, Grace politely informs her, while wrenching herself from her grip, "*I don't want the yellow drops! Noooooooooooooo!*" Rebecca puts in a *Dumbo* video and calls the drops "raindrops." It works.

Once the drops have had time to work, in comes Rabiah. We all say hello as he opens a drawerful of lenses. Off go the overhead lights. His coal-miner ophthalmoscope makes Gracie laugh when he flicks on its beam. It's the moment of truth. He wheels his chair up good and close, takes hold of her face, peers into her eye, looks around. We watch him, watch Gracie . . .

"Looks good and healthy in here."

We exhale. On the monitor next to *Dumbo*, an eye chart for kids who can't read yet appears. Rabiah covers Grace's left eye, asking her to tell him what she sees.

"Your hand," Gracie says.

Now *he* laughs. "Over here, on the screen."

"A chick."

"Now?"

"A house . . . a boat . . . a car . . . a phone."

To test depth of field, he slides some high-tech lenses in over-size black frames onto her face. "Can you grab the fly's wings?"

She reaches out, tries to.

"Which animals are popping up at you?"

She gets those right as well.

"Which of the circles?"

After a few minutes more of the same, he tells us, "Excellent." Turning back to Grace: "Okay, you're all done." He gives her a pat as she hops into Jennifer's lap.

"Everything looks good. There are two scars in her cornea, but they won't affect her vision because they aren't centered over the lens. She was lucky. The ocular pressure in both eyes is normal. Both eyeballs are round, firm, and normal."

Grinning like a couple of morons, we hold Grace and blubber

our thanks. She has 20/20 vision in the right eye, he tells us, 20/15 in the left "because of all the extra work it's been doing."

Peter K. Rabiah is officially and forever The Man. The more enthusiastically we communicate this to him, the more embarrassed he becomes, which just makes him more of The Man. Whatever primitive justice "an eye for an eye" brings about, this dear fellow provides something more evolved. Jennifer's gratitude is so overwhelming that, once he steps out to respond to a nurse's question, she suggests that she "would do anything for the guy," up to and including "you know . . ."

In the fifteen years I've known her, this is the first time she's gone here, at least in a way that didn't make it clear she was kidding.

"He doesn't wear a ring," she points out.

She's giddy. I'm giddy. Rabiah's still out of earshot, we hope. We're taking turns hugging our daughter, telling her how brave she has been, what a great job she did of getting all better. Yeah, yeah, I can see, is her attitude. She wants to watch *Dumbo*, not put on her jacket.

Says Mommy, "I just thought . . ."

Say what? Is she serious? "What about a case of Cristal?"

"Yeah, that too."

Like every red-blooded wife, Jennifer has a shortlist of mostly tall men she has a theoretical dispensation to spend one, but only one, night with: Michael Jordan, Bruce Springsteen, Barack Obama, Tom Hanks, David Letterman. The usual suspects for women her age, all the more unthreatening to me because of their remoteness. Dr. Rabiah's different. He really couldn't be much more present, and it's apparently relevant that he seems to be straight and unmarried. And talk about status in Jennifer's eyes! The man restored our baby's vision. Grace's clear, huge, long-lashed, and flashing blue eye had been damaged, perhaps beyond repair; he repaired it. Our insurance will cover all but about $200 of the total bill. (Our co-payments are $15 per office visit, $30 for specialists.) But clearly we owe Peter Rabiah much more than money. C'mon, don't we owe him at least a Jenny Special? Much to my nervous astonishment, the idea doesn't seem *that* preposterous.

That was six weeks ago. Grace's eye has never worked or looked better, and everyone's eternally grateful. We forgot about suing the wand manufacturer. Jennifer's feeling pretty proud of herself for getting us through the ordeal. Grace returned to school, to the park, to ballet class; she hosts and goes on play dates, and is just about ready to lose her training wheels.

But so—did it happen? Preposterous is as preposterous does, if you know what I'm saying. Has my frisky comedienne repaid her knight in shining armor the most generous way she knows how? Between the half dozen office visits, all the time I've spent out of town on the book tour and poker circuit, and the fact that "Peter" lives only three towns away, she certainly *could* have. I would think that I'd know if it happened, but even then I could never be certain. And which would be worse: not knowing it happened, or believing it did when it didn't?

As Yogi Berra reminds us, you can observe a lot of things just by watching. I'm home for another eleven days before heading to Vegas for the final two weeks of the World Series of Poker, and I'd like to find out before then. So after our daughters are safely tucked in, I deploy four and half decades of poker acumen by watching their mother's green eyes as I ever so casually ask, "How're things with our pal Dr. Rabiah?"

Pregnant pause, during which I remind myself that Penelope waited to tell Odysseus of "all she'd borne at home" until after he slaughtered the suitors, identified who had carved their headboard, got himself cleaned up and settled in for the evening. Only then does *he* admit to Circe's "deceits and magic," though not to subduing that kinky enchantress in the biblical sense. All he tells his wife of Calypso is that the golden-haired, eternally youthful nymph(o) with an island-size dungeon "detained him there"—for seven years!—"but he held out against her," which while the *case* ain't exactly the truth. (Want the truth? *YOU CAN'T HANDLE THE TRUTH!!!*) The superfine Phaeacian princess Nausicaa, before whom Odysseus appeared on the beach *buck naked*, just doesn't come up in the marriage bed at Ithaca; nor do his camp wives on the plain outside Troy. No, what Odysseus tells Penelope is the version of his road trip he knows she wants to hear, which is why they lived happily ever after, at least until Dante caught up with them. Penelope's version of events at home is that, with eligible suitors galore and her husband presumably dead, she remained *aglaopistos* (Homeric Greek for "110 percent committed") to her wily husband every last minute of his twenty-year swath across Mediterranean womanhood.

Jennifer's version is a grin and a shrug, then a wink. We stare at each other, not speaking. *I'm really sorry, sweetheart, but there's been a misunderstanding. The doctor only said I have acute angina.* I smile, try to smile, but I'm bluffing. Following Rabiah's detailed instructions, she has nursed Gracie's eye back to life. Yeah, but what else did she do? I feel rage and abject curiosity, stupendously lucky and grateful, but I give her my steeliest poker face. *And?* She stretches and yawns, looking comely as hell, but I still don't have clue number one about what to say, what to do, as she moseys down the hall toward our bedroom.

HEY McMORON

In this context there's no disrespect
so when I bust my rhyme, you break your necks . . .
Let's get ill, that's the deal.

      —BLACK EYED PEAS, "Let's Get It Started"

Be courteous and friendly: No one likes a whiner . . .
Don't give a player advice in the middle of a hand even if he asks for it.

      —RICHARD D. HARROCH and LOU KRIEGER, *Poker for Dummies*

On May 18, 2004, after providing some personal cases in point for my friend Andy Glazer as he worked on *The Complete Idiot's Guide to Poker*, I finished fourth in the WSOP limit hold'em championship at Binion's Horseshoe. During the televised final-table action, a medium-size wrangle broke out between me and Ellix Powers, a player from Los Angeles. Ellix had been taunting T. J. Cloutier and David Chiu, two of the greatest players alive. Referring to one of T.J.'s second-place finishes, for example, Ellix repeatedly told him, "You can't close," this despite T.J.'s having won the *previous* WSOP tournament, not to mention about sixty other major championships and, oh yeah, a *pair* of Player of the Year bracelets. And despite the fact that runner-up is a lucrative accomplishment itself, especially now that tournament fields routinely number in the thousands. And no, Ellix wasn't taunting *me*, in case you're wondering; he was putting it to the biggest kahunas in classic hari-kiri fashion. *Speaking truth to power* is what this pseudo-David-and-Goliath BS is often called, except that what was coming out of Ellix's mouth was demonstrably, *phosphorescently* false. T.J., a lethal weapon disguised as a sixty-five-year-old poker player, chose not to waste energy or dignity responding to Ellix on camera. Ellix, being Ellix, took this as encouragement to keep right on woofin'.

Finally, after Ellix had bet in the dark (without looking at his hand, that is, or without waiting to see the next card) for the two-dozenth time, I told him, "You're disrespecting the game." Clearly surprised, in no small part because I wasn't even in the hand against him, he fixed his vibrating pupils on me and maintained that he had every right to bet dark. I couldn't disagree with that, but I said he was missing the point.

Ellix finally got me so rattled that a few hands later I called him down holding only a queen-high, a donkey mistake costing me several thousand more chips, though I eventually won more of Ellix's chips than he won of mine. He eliminated some very tough hombres, however, and took tiger-shark bites out of Todd Brunson, An "the Boss" Tran, Patty Gallagher, Oslo's Jan "the Balrog" Sjavik, and me.

Johnny "World" Hennigan had tongue planted stiffly in cheek when he defended Ellix on camera, saying, "He's good for poker." But mostly Johnny World laughed at and with Ellix, which is what I should've done. This is how Hennigan's deceptively goofy sense of humor works—along with "World Class,"

he was deferentially called "Flakes" in his hometown of Philly—
and it has served him well in countless high-stakes confrontations
on poker and pool tables, where he uses it to cool his opponents.
An integral part of his hustle, it's also just the way he is. The bottom line is that Hennigan had a huge chip lead when Ellix began
to get crazy, and anything that disrupted the rhythm of opponents playing catch-up gave Johnny World more of an edge. He
eventually won the event, with the Boss finishing second, Patty
third, Ellix seventh.

But I didn't tell Ellix he was disrespecting the game simply
because he bet dark. And the last thing I wanted was to get into a
distracting beef at a televised WSOP final table. I was trying to
win the damn thing, not enforce poker etiquette. Plus you *want*
your opponents to put money in the pot with as little information as possible. Another factor I considered was that Ellix was a
recently homeless African American, with lengthy gray dreads
and a streetwise comportment; I'm a buzz-cut loaf of Kenilworth
white bread given to professorial airs. Whether this was relevant
the television gods only knew; they also could edit the tape so
that context flew right out the window. But Ellix was 186,000
miles out of line, in my opinion, and I couldn't bite my tongue
any longer. Then, instead of leaving our fairly ugly exchange on
the cutting-room floor, ESPN featured it in its broadcast, even
counting down to it dozens of times as the No. 2 Moment of the
'04 World Series. That's entertainment, I guess.

As the incident was played and replayed, I had my defenders
on the poker circuit and out there in cyberspace, but I also got to
read plenty of the following: "When McManus said 'Poker is a
beautiful game,' I couldn't stop laughing. I mean, it is a great
game, but saying that just makes you sound like a tool." "I love

McManus' book . . . but he came off like a pompous ass last night screaming about the sanctity of the game. It felt like the ramblings of baseball nutjobs who still scream about the DH." (Nota bene: Nutjob, pompous ass, and laughable tool certainly, but the videotape reveals that not only did I not scream, I didn't even raise my darn voice. Didn't say "sanctity," either.) "I just think Jim 'Mr. Best-Seller' McManus needs to get over himself. He gets mad at Ellix for raising in the dark, then calls it, loses the hand, and blames Ellix? Hey McMoron, Ellix wasn't the one who put your chips in the pot." *Ouch!* But in the interest of fairness and balance, I'll see all these guys in the No Spin Zone at eight and eleven eastern (check local listings), then we'll "take it outside" the ESPN Zone over on Broadway and Forty-second. Or we'll blog ourselves into a stupor. In the meantime, let's give the last word to Andrew N. S. Glazer, the unchallenged dean of tournament reporters: "Because Powers's game was so unusual and unpredictable, he was throwing off everyone else; standards were changing, and players were making calls and raises with hands they would never normally have considered even playing, much less attacking with. Say what you will about how many floors his mind's personal elevator stops at, Ellix Powers's approach threw some of the world's finest off balance, and he played fearlessly." No, changed my mind. Last word goes to the Ellixir, who earned it by telling an ESPN correspondent, "I've been a poor man all my life. The [$40,040 in prize] money is cool. There's always tomorrow. God bless all of you."

In other WSOP news: On May 22, minutes before the $10,000 no-limit hold'em championship got under way, Andy and I made a friendly little last-longer bet—whoever went out first paid the other guy twenty bucks. Poor Andy, who wasn't feeling well to begin with, caught a run of cold cards, played them like a mule, and lasted less than four hours, comfortably winning our wager by 135 minutes.

Six weeks later, with Fourth of July fireworks going off in the night sky over Los Angeles, Andy died in his house up in Hollywood. The papers originally said "from complications caused by a blood clot," but some of his neighbors in L.A. told me it was from a self-inflicted gunshot, and the coroner confirmed it. Andy had struck me and others as something of a hypochondriac, but he was genuinely addicted to red meat, starchy food, and painkillers, this combined with insomnia (later diagnosed as apnea), bad luck in love, type 2 diabetes, a pronounced tendency toward depression, and other health issues. His romance and weight problems exacerbated each other as well as the diabetes, as well as the apnea, as well as the depression, and for a while he mixed sleeping pills with painkillers. He also kept guns in the house. As the spiral got out of control, he tried a night breathing mask for his apnea, and that seemed to help. Andy went six five, two eighty, dimensions you might not expect from his nimble prose. He'd become, at forty-eight, one of poker's deepest thinking, most culturally astute writers and by far its best tournament reporter: accurate, punny, voluminous, tactically insightful, speedy to post on the Internet, scorchingly honest when his latest home site gave its blessing. (He often insisted that his middle initials stood for No Shit.) But the best was yet to come, we all thought. The poker world misses him terribly.

Besides Andy's manuscript, I'd packed Don Hensrud's *Mayo Clinic on Healthy Weight* for my trips to L.A. and Las Vegas, though Don's remains a book I haven't been able to profit from.

But at least I'm not alone in ignoring sound advice about eating habits. Nope, we're talkin' 'bout 43 percent of my generation, baby. Out of seventy-five million American boomers, a poll indicated that about thirty-five million of us would rather eat what we want *even if it would kill us within ten years.*

When I go out of town to play tournaments, however, I always shrink a belt notch or two. The reasons are obvious and plentiful: no Sub-Zero access, no thirds of Jennifer's cooking, and because of the stakes we play for, I drink almost nothing. Instead of sitting on the couch after dinner, I'm sitting at the poker table—sitting up, tense but sober, not scarfing more food down my throat.

Poker trips cost me in other ways, though, mainly because I lose money in four fifths of these dadburn events. On top of travel and hotel expenses and the 6–15 percent juice the promoters scruze out, you pay 40 percent in state and federal taxes on prize money, on top of which you're expected to tip. It's a racket, this poker boom, damn it. Even if you manage to keep your bankroll in the black, the physical toll catches up with you. Full-time tournament rounders can lounge abed till the crack of noon (or later) every day, while players with nonpoker jobs have to tumble through endlessly upside-down sleep cycles. Most of the Legends of Poker events at the Bicycle Club, for example, begin at 7:15 p.m. Pacific time, 9:15 on my body clock. Last August I was lucky enough to make the final table in the first event I played after flying in that afternoon, so I didn't get eliminated until 8—that is, 10—the next morning. For the next nine days I went to bed at 6 a.m. on average and got up around 2, which was fine while the tournament lasted. Yet flying home on September 3, I had to readjust overnight to family and teaching hours on central time. *Boo-hoo-hoo-hoo-hoo-hoooooooooooooo!*

But however voluntary and fun my routine is, repeating this jet-lag-squared pattern more or less monthly can't be good for my digestion, sleep, exercise regimen, or ability to concentrate, particularly as I get older. Circadian timekeeping in the hypothalamus is critical to all higher forms of life, from insects on up. Human motherboards have a built-in pacemaker called the suprachiasmatic nucleus that regulates the firing of electrical synapses in our nervous system and the metabolism of sugars and fats. Tilt your SCN back and forth a few times too often, and you'll get frazzled, fat, sleepy, and dumb pretty quick. And once you're past fifty, you especially don't want to put too much stress on it, for much the same reason that you wouldn't let your supercalifragilisticexpialidocious valve get obstructed. Then there's the serious-as-a-heart-attack fact that more strokes and myocardial infarctions occur in the morning than at any other time of day, whereas vitality peaks in the late afternoon. Intelligent people schedule themselves accordingly. But what are a.m. and p.m. any more, actuaries might well inquire, for McMoron or Professor McManus?

And is it George Bush's fault that I've yet to schedule an appointment to get my bloodwork done? Because I seem to recall Drs. Gau and Hensrud and Martin telling me to have my liver enzymes, cholesterol, and triglycerides checked within ninety days of my physical. *That was two years ago, fella.* Gau and Hensrud, I know, have been counting on me to follow up with Lynn Martin. If she or I have any questions, they stand ready to answer them, but they're not gonna hound me to behave like a responsible adult. I haven't even weighed myself once, though judging by belt notches I'm about where I was in August '02.

"Dear Subscriber," said the e-mail, "Fall is unofficially here, and the chilly weather and shorter days may leave you tempted to curl up on the toasty couch in front of the television with a nice bag of chips. Your heart may have a thing or two to say about that, though. And as former President Clinton has discovered, taking care of your heart is vitally important. Find out what bypass surgery means and how cholesterol drugs can help protect your heart." The letter was dated September 8, 2004, and signed, "Sincerely, Mayo.Clinic.com."

Dear Mayo.Clinic.com, I was tempted to write, I've never liked chips or French fries, though it takes five wild horses to keep me from eating just about any other form of potato. I also tend not to "curl up," on the couch or anywhere else. And I've never needed the excuse of chilly weather or seductive TV to overeat in the evening. Come rain or come shine, I do that most days of the year.

But I did get the point of the letter. I also appreciated that the folks up in Rochester were still looking out for me. I even liked their tone of address: warm, fuzzy, topical, practical. If you can't control the fats in your blood with diet, drugs, and exercise, we'll be happy to saw through your ribs and reroute a few things, maybe borrow a length of pipe from your leg, send you home good as new. Don't you worry!

Let's do it, a part of me said. Splice in some new valves and tubes, cancel my bad habits and family history, recommence with a *cardia rasa*. Even if I didn't always follow their advice, I trusted the Mayo cardiologists and surgeons implicitly. On top of being runner-up on the *U.S. News* list, the whole clinic just exudes a good vibe. At a dinner party that September I was seated beside an oncologist who taught and practiced at the University of Chicago Hospitals, without question one of the most prestigious research institutions around, and a Mayo competitor. We were talking about my physical, cancer families and heart families, Cheney's cardiologist's problems, Leon Kass and Janet Rowley. Though my dinner companion supported Dr. Rowley's position on ES cell research, she still had "a ton" of respect for Dr. Kass. Toward the end of the dessert course, she asked me, "Do you know the three most overrated things on the planet?" I told her I had no idea, though I thought I had a pretty good sense of where our conversation was headed: more support for Leon Kass and Dick Cheney as *people*. I was not even close. "Home cooking," she told me, thoroughly deadpan, "out-of-town sex, and the Mayo Clinic."

Two of my favorite guys have had bypasses now, though neither took place at the Mayo. David Letterman underwent emergency quintuple bypass surgery in January 2000 at New York–Presbyterian, the same hospital Bill Clinton went to for his four years later. Dave had been deadly serious on camera the week before, when he shocked his audience and guest Regis Philbin by announcing he planned to undergo heart tests. His cholesterol level was "borderline," he said, but his father died of a heart attack in his fifties. Referring to himself, he said the worst-case scenario would be to "open daddy's rib cage . . . and I don't want that." But his doctors decided to operate after an angiogram revealed he had a blocked artery. The cardiologist who performed the procedure predicted a rapid recovery. "Dave has the heart muscle of a twenty-year-old," he said, and that made me want to start jogging. I didn't "because of my knees," but at least Dave resparked my intentions.

Upon his return to the show five weeks later, Dave brought his entire medical staff onstage. The normally cryogenic Hoosier got positively weepy while thanking the docs. It was beautiful. Cooling back down on subsequent shows, he said he hoped the stretch of I-465 that detours past Indianapolis would be renamed the Dave Letterman Bypass. A fake Rand McNally map came up on the screen, then a hand-lettered "Dave Letterman Expressway" sign, then a newspaper ad for a strip club off Exit 12B of the Letterman.

Men.

In 2004 it was Clinton's turn. He had just given a rousing speech at the Democratic Convention in Boston. On TV he looked strong, ruddy, clear-sighted; he was only fifty-eight, after all. We knew he'd given up cheeseburgers and started to jog while he was in the White House, and every time I saw him on television or in photographs he seemed to be in wonderful shape.

But after experiencing mild chest pain and shortness of breath, he went to the hospital on September 3. In keeping with the new openness about health problems, especially when cases in point can be driven home as a public service, we were told that an angiogram revealed blockages in some of the former president's coronary arteries. Journalists reminded us that when he left office in 2001, his cholesterol level was at 233 milligrams per deciliter, above the upper edge of normal, and that his bad LDL had jumped forty points to 177 during the last year of his presidency. In a marvelously candid presurgery telephone interview with Larry King, Clinton admitted, "I've had some difficulty ever since I got out of the White House in getting my distance up in running. And I just had a feeling a couple of days ago I had to have it checked, when I finally got some tightness in my chest. And I hadn't done any exercise. That's the first time that ever happened to me." He said he'd stopped taking Zocor because he'd gotten his cholesterol level "down low." (Had I taken my Zocor that morning? I had.) "Some of this is genetic, and I may have done some damage in those years when I was too careless about what I ate." Without the surgery, he said, "there is virtually a hundred percent chance I'll have a heart attack."

On Labor Day, about sixty hours after his checkup, he underwent a quadruple coronary artery bypass. The operation began at 8 a.m. and was over by noon. At 4:30 p.m., doctors spoke with reporters, saying that Clinton was awake but still sedated and on a ventilator. The docs and reporters described the procedure to us. Once you're anesthetized, a breathing tube is inserted through your mouth. This tube is attached to a ventilator, which breathes for you during the surgery. You're unable to speak, but you can communicate with notes and hand gestures. *Help! Three hundred million people are watching my chest get ripped open!* Some of the reporters were also M.D.'s and able to be quite specific. Most coronary bypasses, we learned, involve a long incision right down the center of the chest. The surgeon cuts the breastbone down the middle and opens the rib cage to expose the heart.

One surgical method stops the patient's heart; the other is performed on a beating heart. Clinton had the former procedure because it was deemed safest for his vascular condition. While a pump oxygenated and circulated his blood, healthy blood vessels were taken from the wall of his chest, as well as from his leg, and then stitched in to bypass clogged vessels. (Try *that* at Lourdes, I thought, or in Al Qaeda's highest-rated infirmary.) Vein grafts become clogged much more quickly than artery grafts, and the patient winds up needing repeat operations or angioplasties. While arteries are preferred for the grafts, since each person has a limited supply of suitable arteries, doctors often need to—*enough!* It was all unbelievably important, but the psychosomatic symptoms were killing me.

During his September 8 monologue, Letterman fired away at his old favorite target. "Clinton had bypass surgery on Monday after undergoing some tests last week. Now hundreds are lining up outside their doctor's office looking for the same tests to be conducted on them. Clinton has that effect on people. In fact, back in '98 during the impeachment hearings, hundreds got in line waiting for oral sex." Rimshot, groan, flat clash of cymbals. A few nights later, Dave had a new variation. "Former President Bill Clinton had quadruple bypass heart surgery last week. Apparently Al Gore had a similar procedure. About four years ago, he had what is called an Oval Office bypass." That Dave had undergone the same surgery made his sexual-mortal-political entendres seven times funnier, I thought. As with most humor, though, the more I analyzed it, the less funny it got. So *that* was how Bush became president.

Good for Dave. Good for Bill. And I now understood who was next. Bypasses are fairly routine these days, with more than 300,000 conducted each year. Surely my numbers, should I ever get the follow-up blood panels, would point straight in that direction. I even looked forward to it, in a way. Get it over with once and for all.

Feeling twinges to the left of my breastbone, I Googled with a new sense of purpose the *U.S. News & World Report* listing the Cleveland Clinic as the best place in the country to have this procedure. The second-best place was the Mayo; third best was Duke University. New York–Presbyterian, where the comedian and the president had theirs, was No. 7, and both those guys seem to be fine. (New York–Pres had a death rate of 3.93 percent for coronary bypasses performed in 2001, higher than the 2.18 percent overall for the thirty-five hospitals in the state that perform them.) As the twinges became more intense, I scanned down the *U.S. News* rankings. My God! In Chicago, Loyola University Hospital came in at No. 25, with Lutheran General hanging tough at No. 36. Northwestern Memorial, where Cigna would want me to go, was No. 43. Out of 50. If testing determined I needed a bypass, I'd have to wheedle an assignment to go back up to Rochester, tear open my shirt, and throw myself at Gerald Gau's mercy.

A few weeks after Clinton's surgery, Dick Cheney experienced shortness of breath and was taken for tests to George Washington University Hospital. We were told that his EKG was normal, that a readout of his pacemaker—that is, of the cardioverter defibrillator implanted in his chest—showed that it hadn't been activated, indicating that his heart rate hadn't fluctuated. The sixty-three-year-old vice president had had four heart attacks, the first when he was thirty-seven. After his fourth, on November 22, 2000—the thirty-seventh anniversary of JFK's assassination, as the chads were being scrutinized and the Dade County votes re-re-recounted—Cheney said he would finally quit smoking, watch his diet, and begin regular daily exercises on a treadmill. A man after my own heart, I'm afraid, though mine's lower tip points to the left.

As if all this heart business weren't mortifying enough, I found myself trying to read *How We Die*, Sherwin Nuland's lurid account of the half dozen most common ways that Americans purchase the farm. But the best I could do was gingerly scan a few pages, so graphic were Nuland's descriptions. In the fateful year of 1951, for example, the author is a third-year med student. The first patient he ever treats by himself is one James McCarty, a sedentary, meat-loving fifty-two-year-old Irish American smoker complaining of chest pains. Reading this, of course, triggers more than one jumpy double take: James McWho? It gets worse— much, much worse. Because at the very moment young Dr. Nuland sits down at his new patient's bedside, McCarty-McManus "suddenly threw his head back and bellowed out a wordless roar that seemed to rise up out of his throat from somewhere deep within his stricken heart. He hit his balled fists with startling force against the front of his chest in a single synchronous thump, just as his face and neck, in the flash of an instant, turned swollen and purple." Swollen and purple, huh? *Roaring?* So much for my cherished idea of a stab of discomfort followed by moderate throat clearing. I cringe and read on: "His eyes seemed to have pushed themselves forward in one bulging thrust, as though they were trying to leap out of his head. He took one immensely long, gurgling breath, and died." Less than two paragraphs into the book and James McWhatever has already expired in mind-bending agony. But the insult to James isn't over. Far from it. Closed-chest cardiopulmonary resuscitation has yet to be invented, so the neophyte doctor decides to intervene the best way he knows how. "I made a long incision starting just below the left nipple, from McCarty's breastbone around as far back as—" Christ! Yet how am I supposed to think clearly about my own heart's well-being if I can't even follow a few lines of text? Wincing, averting my eyes, I force myself to scan a bit further: "Another long cut through the bloodless muscle . . . slipped [the retractor] in between the ribs, and turned its ratchet just far enough to allow my hand to squeeze inside and grasp—" *Basta!* But even a tentative glance down the page reveals that grasping this poor Irish beefeater's heart is "like holding in one's palm a wet, jellylike bagful of hyperactive worms . . ." By this point, of course, a clammy hand clutches *my* ventricles, massaging the chambers so vigorously I think I might vomit. Yet this is no bloodthirsty account by a gore-obsessed schlockmeister. Nor is it Buñuel and Dalí slicing a cow's eyeball in *An Andalusian Dog* for grisly postmodern effect. *How We Die* is the National Book Award–winning prose of a gifted professor of both surgery and the history of medicine at Yale, for God's sake, *a place where they spread lots of hold'em.* Any self-respecting secular humanist should be able to stomach Dr. Nuland's lucid account of a run-of-the-mill myocardial infarction, yet I skim till he changes the subject.

Back in my nonreading life, I picked up what I thought was the flu and/or bronchitis, probably on a flight from L.A. No flu vaccine had been available that fall, and I cursed all and sundry— Chiron, the FDA, Bush, Cheney, Halliburton, the Tyrell Corporation, the moron coughing in the seat behind me, the inconsiderate sneezers up in first class, with whom I was forced to share a ventilation system—for how awful I felt. But I wasn't experiencing anything worse than the occasional twinge in my chest, which I put down to all the damn coughing. Even so, on October 23, 2004, I decided to go in for a checkup.

NO SCHMUTZ IN *HERE*

What are the hopes of Man? Old Egypt's King
    Cheops erected the first pyramid,
And largest, thinking it was just the thing
    To keep his memory whole and mummy hid;
But somebody or other rummaging,
    Burglariously broke his coffin's lid.

                —BYRON, *Don Juan*, Canto I, CCXIX

Throw up a finga if ya feel the same way
Dre puttin' it down for Californ-i-a

    —2PAC, featuring Dr. Dre, "California Love"

When I call for an appointment, Lynn Martin's office insists that I provide them with hepatic and lipid (liver and cholesterol) panels before I see a doctor, so what can I say? I don't drink that evening, eat extra salad, and forgo dessert. Before breakfast the next morning, I go in, make a fist, and surrender enough blood through my right antecubital for any test they might wanna run.

Dr. Martin has no open slots, so I wind up being seen the next day by my old friend Dennis Hughes. He whirls in, sits at the tiny desk in the corner of the examining room, and starts reading and typing into my e-file. Corduroy jeans under his lab coat and tie, a few days of stubble, brown hair sticking up like he just yanked off a stocking cap. Huck Finn, M.D. The panel results aren't back yet, but the nurse has already taken my temperature, blood pressure, and heart rate and entered them into the file. After 6.2 seconds of bedside manner, Hughes asks, "So what are your symptoms?"

"I think I got the flu on a plane, either that or from one of my kids."

"At this time of year they bring something new home from school every day."

We agree. "I've been hacking for a couple of weeks. Maybe a couple of twinges—"

"Are you smoking?"

"Haven't had a cigarette in over five years."

"That's good. Keep that up."

"I will."

"That's important." A pause. Is my nose getting longer? "Any history of asthma?"

"Nope."

"Noticed any flecks of blood in what you're bringing up?"

As I shake my head no, he moves behind me and listens to my chest: front, back, left, right. Tap, tap, tap. Thump. Upper, lower. Moving the stethoscope around, he asks me to breathe normally, then to take a deep breath and hold it. As he listens and probes, he's bearing in mind several factors, which he later types up. My temperature is 98.4. I'm alert, oriented, comfortable. My eyes are anicteric, with no conjunctival injection, EOMI or PERRL. My ears have normal bilateral EACs and TMs. My nares have no purulent rhinorrhea. No nasal polyps or septal deviation. In terms of my oropharynx: no erythema, tonsillar exudates, or mass. My neck has a normal range of motion. No thyromegaly. No bruits. No cervical adenopathy, meaning no abnormal lymph nodes in my neck. My heart rate sounds fine, without murmur. My lungs have decreased breath sounds and rales in the right base. Good air movement, however. Dr. Hughes's formal impression? Could be mucous plugging with atelectasis, or else it's pneumonia. "Sounds like you have either pertussis or pneumonia," is how he puts it in Patient English.

"Pertussis?"

"Yes. Whooping cough."

Damn. "What were you hearing, exactly?"

"Rales." Anticipating my next question, he adds, "A bubbling or crackling sound. Rales on one side of the chest suggest pneumonia. When I tapped your chest, I was listening for a dull thud instead of a hollow drumlike sound."

"Would this be called walking pneumonia?"

He snickers at that, though he does keep it subtle, God bless him.

"You know, since I'm walking and flying around with it."

He nods, shakes his head. What I should ask him is, "I *amuse* you? I make you *whoop* with laughter?" But I don't. I'm neither packing blue steel nor in any kind of position to antagonize Huck here. Because he's a made guy and I'm not.

"The term," he says, turning around, with the merest picogram of amusement, "may have referred to the fact that it's treatable outside the hospital." Then back to the keyboard and screen. "There's been an epidemic of pertussis around here this fall, and you have some of the symptoms. This virus usually strikes young children, but lately it's been turning up in their parents."

I make mental notes to tell Jennifer to Google pertussis: symptoms in children, ways to avoid. My impression is, Hughes is convinced I don't have it.

We'll see. Getting down to business, he directs me a couple of miles away to the radiology department of Glenbrook Hospital, where Gracie met Rabiah on Friday the 13th. Moving at the speed of light, Order #33848919 XRAY CHEST FRONTAL & LATERAL beats me there by a good fifteen minutes. Hughes has asked for a wet reading—so-called from the days when X rays, not to mention patients, got hung up for hours or weekends while the processing chemicals dried—and for the results to be immediately phoned in to him. A friendly technician named Maya positions me against the silvery grid, leaves the room, comes back to reposition me, leaves the room, then comes back to say I'm all done. Four minutes later the receptionist hands me a phone: Dr. Hughes. I have pneumonia, he says. He recommends that I take a new antibiotic called Levaquin, so powerful that I'll need only one 750 mg capsule per day, for five days. I don't ask whether I might be allergic, assuming he'll know this from having my file on his screen. I just thank him. He e-mails the scrip to our Walgreens, and it's ready when I get to the pharmacy ten minutes later. Even with our Cigna co-payment, the five pills cost thirty dollars, which inspires in me extra faith that they'll work: a market-based variation on the placebo effect. I also buy a pair of $6.99 gray felt slippers, since these might help too. Grandma Grace prescribed them 11/26/58, to be worn till I'm snugly tucked in and have said all my prayers, Order #02271947. Still good.

I won't see the X-ray results printed out for another week or so, but the wet reading that the radiologist, Jonathan Berlin, zipped back to Hughes read, "Frontal and lateral views of the chest dated 10/25/04 demonstrate focal alveolar airspace disease in the right lower lobe. In this patient with history of cough, this most likely relates to right lower lobe pneumonia . . . Due to the fact that an underlying pulmonary lesion cannot be completely excluded, follow-up frontal and lateral plain films of the chest in 6 weeks are recommended to confirm resolution." Just like I figured: walking focal alveolar airspace disease.

Because of the educated and well-equipped efficiency of Dennis, Maya, Jonathan, and colleagues, the toastiness of the slippers (or "slippy-socks," as Grandma Grace called them), and the targeted potency of Levaquin, I got to recover at home, where I work. I was lucky. About 1.2 million Americans are hospitalized each year for pneumonia, the third most frequent reason. (Births are first, heart disease next.) Pneumonia is tied with influenza as our sixth leading cause of death; if I died now, the tie would be broken. Symptoms include fever, cough, shortness of breath, headache, muscle pain, fatigue, gastrointestinal distress, and mental confusion. Check, check, check, check, check, check, check, and check. Shortness? Check. Spare tire? Check. Plus pneumonia hits old farts much harder, and this is my new demographic. (David Sedaris, a man five years, nine months, and four days younger than I, referred to himself as "elderly" in *The New Yorker*, and we all know how vigilant its fact checkers are.) Elderly pneumoniacs have lower survival rates, particularly those with other medical problems. It's how people with heart problems go out if they know what's good for them. "A blessing," their families are told. As opposed to what James McCarty, Grandpa

Jim, Grandma Grace, Grandma Betsy, and my father went through . . .

You tend to get pneumonia when your defense system is weakened by an upper respiratory tract viral infection or a case of the flu. When antibiotics don't kill it and it doesn't kill *you*, it can lead to abscesses—thick-walled, pus-filled cavities that form when the infection destroys lung tissue. Left untreated, abscesses cause hemorrhages in the lung, but antibiotics have made these less likely. Long live the makers of Levaquin!

Airway checkpoints normally protect our lungs from bacteria and other microbes. Larger particles get filtered out in the nose—especially an elderly male nose, with all those extra hairs. When smaller ones manage to sneak through, sensors in the nasal passages trigger coughing or sneezing, which drives most alien particles back out where they came from. Even if they're stealthy enough to reach the bronchioles deep in our lungs, nearly all will be trapped in a balmy mucous blanket and recycled upward and out by the beating movements of tiny hairlike cells called cilia, part of what doctors call the mucociliary escalator. (Non-M.D. snifflers routinely misidentify it, of course, as the mucociliary *elev*ator, the mucoconciliatory lift, the hock chute, the icky green blanky, or the translucent booger express.) Bacteria and other infectious agents that evade the cilia are attacked in the immune system's alveolar sacs by microphages, large white blood cells that literally eat foreign particles, but snafus occur down here as well. You can not only wind up with bronchitis, pertussis, a cold, or pneumonia, but sometimes, as in Bridget's case, the immune system attacks the body's own islets of Langerhans, mistaking them for bovine serum albumin, resulting in juvenile diabetes. With

MS, the misguided attack targets the central nervous system. With lupus, it's various organs, usually in girls or young women. In rheumatoid arthritis, the friendly fire of Operation Microbic Freedom destroys cartilage and the lining of the joints. When someone is infected with HIV, the entire immune system is at risk to break down. All of these maladies, however, might be cured by means of embryonic stem cell research.

The Levaquin Dr. Hughes put me on had been approved by the FDA only a few months earlier for treating what is called community-acquired (as opposed to the much more deadly hospital-acquired) pneumonia, so Huck had kept up with the literature. If I'd recently been hospitalized and a sputum culture indicated I had HAP, he would have—what, rushed me to the hospital? Anyway, the World Health Organization was also enthusiastic about Ortho-McNeil's new star anti-infective. "In an effort to address bacterial resistance, the WHO Antimicrobial Resistance Guidelines have called for aggressive, short courses of therapy," reported WHO's spokesman. "Levaquin 750 mg meets these guidelines because it is highly efficacious, well tolerated, and treats CAP in half the time of the standard 500 mg regimen." The tablets are terra-cotta pink for the 250 mg tablet, peach for the 500 mg, and white for my 750 mg horse pills. Such concentration leads to 25 percent less exposure to the drug over the course of treatment and thus helps prevent resistance caused by antibiotic overexposure. The most common side effects of the 750 mg dosage are nausea, diarrhea, itching, abdominal pain, rash, dizziness, and flatulence. Amazingly, ruptures of the shoulder, hand, and Achilles tendons had been reported in takers of Levaquin. It had also been "associated with" the development of phototoxicity ("blistering sunburns," according to the fact sheet) following exposure to sunlight or stints in a tanning salon. Convulsions, tremors, restlessness, anxiety, light-headedness, confusion, hallucinations, paranoia, depression, nightmares, and insomnia were all in the cards, though unlikely. Suicidal thoughts or acts could not be ruled out altogether, the fact sheet was forced to admit.

Three Levaquins into the regimen, I felt 109 percent better. No suicidal itch or pink elephants, both Achilles tendons intact, much less hacking, no flatulence or confusion to speak of— or no more than usual. Only the usual antibiotic spaciness, ultra-smooth turds, and slight loss of appetite. I was revising the "Hey McMoron" chapter, trying to resist the temptation to quote bloggers who supported me ("You we're right Jim!" "Yeah tell em Mr, Mcmurphy"), when I got a call from Dr. Hughes about my blood tests. My total cholesterol was 143, triglycerides 190, bad LDL cholesterol 86—pretty good. The bad news was that my good HDL was only 18, when we wanted it to be at least 40. Even worse, I had elevated liver enzymes. Something called SGOT was 132, with normal being < 41. My serum glutamic pyruvic transaminase (SGPT) was 232, while normal was < 63. Shit.

He told me to stop taking Zocor, the very drug that had been so effective in reducing my LDL. I also had to stop taking aspirin, which helped keep my blood from clogging my arteries.

"Jeez, what's the plan after that?" I asked, more than a little desperate.

"Get your liver retested in a couple of weeks. Then we'll see."

Oy.

As the presidential campaign hit the home stretch, Mr. Bush kept his lead in the polls. I chose to remain optimistic. The Republican brain trust, after all, was asking voters to buy some insultingly far-fetched ideas. The tax code is fair and creates lots of jobs? It's okay to remain the only first-world country without a national health care program? Gay people are evil and dangerous? Dick Cheney is the most creative and open-minded guy to shape energy policy? The cheerleading C student and business failure who pulled every string to avoid serving under fire is up to the vast complexity of our military, diplomatic, intelligence, and security predicaments? C'mon.

Luckily for Mr. Bush, Karl Rove is his answer man. And when he isn't scarfing down his famous eggies—butter, cream, eggs, and bacon fat scrambled into scrumpdiddleyumptiously thermonukular hypertriglyceridemiac devices—Rove eats hayseed resentment for breakfast. *There, there. We're just folks like you. We have ten thousand times more money than you, but since when does that make any difference? We won't make you feel bad for trusting the clergy more than them pointy-headed scientists and French intellectuals with their fancy war medals, even if that's exactly what our Evil Enemies do. And don't worry, we won't let the queers and feminists get away with destroying this country.* An electorate childish and pious enough to swallow this custard, to fail to reraise in the face of this obvious bluff, deserves whatever blows it will suffer, I reasoned, ignoring the inconvenient fact that my daughters would suffer them too if Bush won. We all deserved better than a scaredy-cat politics in which you could sell any tax code, any war plan, any position on science and industry by making threatening noises about freedom and patriotism or declaring you've prayed on it. How could folks not understand that?

During the campaign, the candidate whose daughter was studying to become a doctor pounded away on health care issues. "The medical discoveries that will come from stem cell research are crucial next steps in humanity's uphill climb," declared Senator Kerry. "If we pursue the limitless potential of our science, and trust that we can use it wisely, we will save millions of lives and earn the gratitude of future generations." In the final days before the election, Kerry stood with parents of children with juvenile diabetes who were also registered Republicans, and accused the president of "turning his back on science in favor of ideology." He received standing ovations when he promised to lift the ban on stem cell studies and more than triple the federal dollars for medical research in general. He referred to an Annenberg poll that found that 64 percent of Americans favor federal funding of ES cell research while 28 percent oppose it. When reporters pressed him on his use of the word *ban*, he didn't suggest they were unpatriotic or against helping sick people; he offered expert testimony from a University of Pennsylvania biology professor. Patricia Labosky stood on the stump with him to acknowledge that, technically, the Bush administration had allowed limited funds to be spent, but only for work on a tiny number of pre-2001 cell lines. As a result, she said, more and more prominent researchers were feeling the need to go abroad. Days before the election, Kerry communications director Stephanie Cutter said stem cell research was "the sleeper issue of the campaign."

M.D.'s weighed in, too. In the final issue of *The New England Journal of Medicine* before November 2, Dr. Jeffrey M. Drazen wrote of the urgency: "The example of a single disease, diabetes, suggests the range of possibilities. Suppose that next week a group announced that it had successfully performed experiments showing that genetically identical pancreatic beta cells could be grown in tissue culture with use of a donor nucleus from a patient and human embryonic stem cells. If our working community of biomedical scientists had experience with this technology, it would probably take three to six months for the findings to be replicated; without the needed laboratory know-how . . . these experiments could take years to complete." Doctors would need to be trained, clinical trials and technology would have to be improved, quality-control measures implemented, patients recruited, beta-cell lines created, cells injected, and patients followed for at least thirty months. "As a conservative estimate, if the fundamental breakthrough at the laboratory level occurred next week, it would be more than five years before there was a stem cell–based cure." If Bush won, we would all have to wait even longer.

I was unhappy but not surprised when it happened. Jennifer began talking to the TV as the count began to go the wrong way, and she took little comfort in the fact that her boyfriend Obama was gonna be one of our senators. "He beat Alan Keyes, for God's sake. What can he accomplish outnumbered like that in D.C.?" She stormed off to look at Canadian real estate Web sites. The average winter temperature in Montreal and the prices in Vancouver, the gorgeous city we'd visited on our honeymoon, calmed her down for a moment. What about Italy, where Bea was conceived? Berlusconi. Or Ireland, the country in which we had fallen in love? "More priest-ridden morons than we've got over here," I suggested. "Which is apparently saying something."

"How did this happen!" she yelled.

"I don't know!"

"I wanna move to the EEC, wherever *that* is . . ."

"Start packing."

"Go buy some euros right now, please."

"I'm going, I'm going . . ."

Some good news: Proposition 71, the California Stem Cell Research and Cures Initiative, passed by eighteen percentage points. Senators Dianne Feinstein and Barbara Boxer had both endorsed it. Financial support came from, among others, Bill Gates, eBay founder Pierre Omidyar, the Juvenile Diabetes Research Foundation, and Robert Klein. No, not the explosion of talent who wrote and performed "Colonoscopy," this generation's new anthem, though he must have supported the measure as well. I'm talking Robert *N.* Klein, the real estate developer, the guy who made the case that more than half of California's families, and by implication more than half of *all* families, are affected by at least one of the diseases thought to be curable by ES cell therapies. In the face of the Bush intransigence, Klein said California "can run a substitute national program." The state already had the biggest pool of academic medical centers and private biotechnology companies anywhere. Even Governor Hummer broke with Bush by supporting it. Lieutenant Governor Cruz Bustamante went further, calling stem cell research "this century's gold rush."

States including New York, New Jersey, Illinois, and Wisconsin are now playing a healthy game of catch-up; others have dug in their heels, assertively moving to quash embryonic stem cell studies. In Massachusetts, both sides of the question are especially well represented, with Harvard's Douglas Melton (two of whose

children have juvenile diabetes) the leading proponent of the research, and Republican governor Mitt Romney (whose wife has
MS, who consulted with Melton while formulating his position,
and who is probably running for president) vowing to establish
civil and criminal penalties for conducting it. Fairly soon, boink-
ing a hundred-cell nucleus a few micrometers to the right or left
could win you a Nobel Prize for curing a dreadful disease and/or
get you locked up not only in Kansas or Texas or Alabama but in
the bluest of commonwealths too. (Instead of a scarlet adulterer's
A embroidered onto the breast pocket of her orange jumpsuit,
a Massachusetts researcher would sport a less puritanical scarlet
abortionist's *A*. This is 2006, after all, not 1647. Governor
Bellingham is no longer calling the shots.) Scientists will continue
to vote with their feet. Jose Cibelli is already an honorary South
Korean. Pediatric neurologist Evan Snyder moved from Harvard
to the Burnham Institute in La Jolla after California enacted a
law in 2002 to protect stem cell research. Like other biomedical
optimists, Snyder likens the new initiative to a slightly more
kindhearted Manhattan Project.

Prop 71 authorized tax-free state bonds to provide an average
of $295 million per year over ten years to support stem cell re-
search at California universities, medical schools, and research fa-
cilities. It has the potential to save the state billions of dollars
through new tax revenues and royalties, and by reducing skyrock-
eting medical costs, already more than $110 billion per annum. If
the research funded leads to cures that reduce costs by only 1 percent, the measure will pay for itself.

In other news from the home of *Ursus californicus* and *Gopherus
agassizi* came Stanford's William Hurlbut, a staunch opponent of

embryo research who is a member of the President's Council on Bioethics. He offered a proposal to encourage scientists to create "the equivalent of" ES cells without destroying embryos. His procedure, called altered nuclear transfer, would engineer a human egg that could generate cells with the curative potential of ES cells but without forming an actual embryo. The technique has never been attempted with human cells, but Hurlbut believes it's feasible. Any method acceptable to fellow conservatives offers hope of a middle ground, Hurlbut argues, and his record as an opponent of embryo research would be key to bridging the gap between the two sides. His biggest challenge will be forming a consensus that the altered mass of cells isn't a human embryo. If Hurlbut's doctored egg developed into anything that might be considered a life, even if it was doomed to die while still microscopic, folks even further to the right would cry murder.

Hurlbut is a Christian who did postdoctoral study in theology and medical ethics. He basically wants to noodge the "moral status as human" line drawn by conservatives on the life continuum a hair to the right, hoping its new coordinates will be meaningful. In the womb, he argues, the appearance of an outer sheath, the trophectoderm, is the first sign a fertilized egg has developed into more than one type of cell. His idea is to not allow the trophectoderm to form properly, so the normal flow of signals will stop; if the vital web of communication within the ball of cells is never established, the entity cannot be called an embryo. He compares the entity to egg cells that begin dividing wildly on their own and can grow into unneeded hair, teeth, or tumors (the dermoid cyst that ate Jennifer's right ovary in 1984, for example). Theologians who have studied these tumors, called teratomas, have agreed that they are not embryos because they lack "integrated organization."

Hurlbut consulted with dozens of biologists, including Douglas Melton at Harvard, as well as Catholic bishops, and brought the idea to the council. Dr. Kass's majority embraced it, but progressives were unconvinced and more than a little annoyed. Writing in *The New England Journal of Medicine* of December 30, 2004, Melton and two other bioethicists concluded: "Hurlbut's argument for the ethical superiority of altered nuclear transfer rests on a flawed scientific assumption. He argues . . . that it is acceptable to destroy a CDX2 mutant embryo but not a normal embryo, because the former has 'no inherent principle of unity, no coherent drive in the direction of the mature human form.' But these are ill-defined concepts with no clear biologic meaning, and an alternative interpretation would be that embryos lacking CDX2 develop normally until CDX2 function is required, at which point they die . . . We see no basis for concluding that [Hurlbut's technique] represents a transition point at which a human embryo acquires moral status." Instead, Melton and his colleagues called the proposal "a distraction from the central issue, which is whether it is morally justifiable to use preimplantation-stage human embryos in the search to understand human biology and cure serious diseases. We believe it to be justified, and the diversion of resources to approaches that offer no scientific benefit merely diminishes the likelihood of success."

And then it became even clearer that therapeutic cloning of ES cells needs to continue. In January 2005, an NIH study at the University of (where else?) California at San Diego found that the lines Mr. Bush set aside for research in 2001 have been contaminated with nonhuman molecules from the culture medium used to grow them. All of these lines are now useless.

Will the president be flexible enough to grasp the meaning of this new information, or will he, as he likes to say, "try not to overthink it"? With no more elections to face, will he maintain his born-again mind-set or take Lincoln's example to heart? *I must study the plain, physical facts of the case, ascertain what is possible, and learn what appears to be wise and right.* I wish I could be optimistic.

Ironically, however the president reacts, the states' rights guaranteed (for now) by the Tenth Amendment—the default position of the Solid South since the 1840s—should allow biomedical research to move forward at close to full speed in the parts of America that would've been pursuing it anyway. Bridget won't have to risk imprisonment in Midland or Abilene to get her islet cells regenerated. She can stay home in Illinois, drive up to Wisconsin, or fly out to one of the coasts.

In the meantime, she's working with a new endocrinologist, who has her on a new kind of insulin and testing regimen. On January 19, Bridget also had an encouraging checkup from her ophthalmologist, Tamara Wyse, a hot blonde who graduated first in and was valedictorian of her med school class at the University of Illinois. "With a history of proliferative diabetic retinopathy in both eyes' status post bilateral panretinal photocoagulation and a vitrectomy on the right eye 10 years ago," wrote Dr. Wyse, "her eye exam remains very stable with no active retinopathy and a very mild epiretinal membrane in the right eye." The more laidback but no less heartening language Dr. Wyse used when examining Bridget's eye was, "No schmutz in *here.*" In other words,

Bridget was hanging tough with her not-easy maintenance regimes, and Kirk Packo's 1995 vitrectomy at Rush-Presbyterian-St. Luke's was no less gleamingly effective than Peter Rabiah's artistry on Grace.

Dr. Packo has invented a number of eye-opening devices that bear his name, including the Adjustable Abrasive Membrane Scraper with Pick. (The do-it-yourself model is on sale all this week at Sharper Image for $79.99.) "I go into surgery," says Packo, "with the attitude of asking if there's a way to do the technique better. Is there something I can do better for my patient?" He serves as the principal investigator for NIH research projects and clinical studies. His *Intraocular Look at Vitreous Surgery* won first place at the American Society of Cataract and Refractive Surgery Film Festival, where distribution-rights competition can be stiffer than at Sundance in January. Lately he's been working with Drs. Alan and Victor Chow to develop the Artificial Silicon Retina, the sort of thing concocted only by prop masters for movies like *Blade Runner* and *Minority Report* until folks like Packo and the Chows got to work. A dozen blind or near-blind patients have already used this invention to see.

Following up on my lung, liver, and cardiac issues, Lynn Martin listens to my chest, reads my vitals, and checks my X-ray results. BP 114/70, pulse 74. To Lynn's eye at least, I appear healthy, alert, in no acute distress. I seem pleasant. My chest is symmetrical, percussion normal, with good diaphragmatic excursion. Lungs clear. Normal breath sounds and PMI. No ergophony, thank God! No lifts, heaves, or thrills. Heart RRR (regular rate and rhythm). No murmurs or gallops. No clicks. No peripheral edema. My abdomen is soft, but in a good way: nontender. No masses, organomegaly, or hernia. She pronounces my pneumonia kaput.

My SGPT is back down to 41, she says. No more Zocor. Stethoscoping my carotids, she hears no bruit. My HDL has risen to 41, where it needs to remain, but my total cholesterol is 258 and my triglycerides are 646 mg/dl. Fuck! She encourages me to lose twenty-five pounds, stick to red wine, and not smoke. (When I began seeing Lynn eleven years ago, she was way over-weight; now she looks like a triathlete, which inspires me when-ever I see her, especially when she wears her white jeans and black sweater that sets off her reddish brown locks, even if the inspira-tion only lasts a few minutes.) To replace the Zocor that was poi-soning my liver, she writes a prescription for Zetia, "a brand-new class of statin," and hands me a month's worth of samples. Would a kiss be appropriate? No, it would not. But a shoulder squeeze, definitely. "Probably not *quite* as effective as Zocor," she tells me, "but more easily tolerated by your liver. That's the trade-off."

I'll take it, for now. But the 10 mg Zetias are these tiny little white racetrack-shaped guys, and I wonder how much punch they can pack. "What if they don't work?"

"We'll probably have to put you on Niaspan, Jim. Let's see where you're at in two months."

In one of the great movie lines, the renegade android Roy Batty (Rutger Hauer) puts his hands around the skull of Eldon Tyrell, the streak of frozen corporate slime who manufactured him, and squeezes: "I want more life, fucker." Unlike me, who have never been south of the equator or west of the international date line, Batty has witnessed attack ships on fire off the shoulder of Orion, *c*-beams aglitter in the dark near Tannhäuser Gate. "All those moments will be lost in time," he laments with his last gulp of oxygen, "like tears in rain. Time . . . to die." Wow. Kudos to Philip K. Dick, screenwriters Hampton Fancher and David Peoples, director Ridley Scott, and to Hauer, who reportedly helped craft these lines and certainly made them immortal. I can only hope to go out with a thirtieth as much fearless poetry and grace, though I wouldn't spare Harrison Ford or know whose money-grubbing skull to implode.

As Michael Corleone puts it with his usual Sub-Zero insight, "Hyman Roth has been dying from the same heart attack for the last twenty years." Their negotiations broke down in Havana (Castro, $2 million), and Roth now has chest pains and shortness of breath. Pushing seventy, emitting little *snics* from his nose every couple of seconds, and looking like he's been camped at death's door for a decade, he still has the chutzpah to say, "What I wouldn't give for *snic* twenty more years."

Twenty, huh, Hyman? Good luck. And I'm sure I will feel the same way, in the end. But I've already had twenty more years than Grandpa Jim got, thirteen more than my brother Kevin, thirty-three more than my son. I haven't been nailed by an aneurysm or a Hummer or a magic wand or dementia or cancer. People including myself keep telling me, "Hey, don't have a heart attack," and so far I've obeyed. Driving in twilight or darkness, jammed in a bottleneck on Michigan Avenue or cruising at *c* past the Tannhäuser Gate, my peripheral vision is still pretty good, mainly because my pigment epithelium hasn't been scorched a few thousand times with a two-hundred-milliwatt laser. I'm ahead of the game. Way ahead.

When I'm feeling even more optimistic, there's a version of an afterlife that somehow doesn't strike me as complete wishful thinking. We can feel pleasure looking back on or forward to something while not physically experiencing it *now*, right? If we can look forward to being remembered after we're dead, we don't need to be present for the anticipatory pleasure to pay off beforehand. In each unit of life since 1865 experienced without slavery and with the benefits of a Union preserved, Abraham Lincoln has afterlife. So does, to a lesser extent, everyone who took part in his good works and days. In this sense, a Lincoln (or Trota or Jeanne d'Arc or Shakespeare or Einstein or Ali or Martin Luther King or any first-rate man or woman) is much more alive than his forgotten contemporaries. Such a person may even be more present than the billions of forgotten souls countable now in a census.

Biologically, we live on in children and grandchildren, nieces and nephews, but the architecture and spirit of a life can be carried forward in plenty of other ways too. Not as a tax deduction, unfortunately, but in photographs, anecdotes, life insurance, trophy cases, recipes, pyramids, biographies, toasts, and good works. The better showing I make for myself until 20whatever, the more afterlife I'll hold on to once half my cremains have been scattered in Jennifer's garden, the other half ensconced in a little saw-grass basket on the mantel above our fireplace. The worse my moral and creative hygiene until then, the deader I'll be when I'm outta here.

The physical world is an interesting place, and I don't wanna leave it. I can't even guarantee I won't bawl hysterically (or conveniently get some religion) when my number is up, assuming I get more than two seconds' notice. My mostly hard, mostly dry-feeling body is actually two-thirds water, I'm told, which may be what makes pneumonia a "blessing," baptism such a comfort, bawling warm tears so cathartic, and drowning reputed to be among the least unpleasant ways to expire.

Now, I don't wanna try to overthink this, but I'm 65 percent hydrogen, 18 percent carbon, 3 percent nitrogen, and something like 1 percent each of calcium and phosphorus, with traces of a dozen other elements, including strontium, vanadium, aluminum, zinc, fluorine, lead, and molybdenum. (Symbol *Mo* for this last one, atomic number 42, atomic weight 95.94. A hard, silvery white metal, often confused with lead and graphite.) Maybe the molybdenum's why I've been feeling so *heavy* of late, not because Jimi's cranked loud in my car with the windows rolled up, till my ears bleed. An essential component of nuclear weaponry at Jaber Ibn Hayan and the Namch'on Chemical Complex, as well as of something *we've* got in the works called—get this—Metal Storm: molybdenum, baby. Tamer explanations of my heaviness: to "run" one mile these days takes me at least thirteen minutes. And the earth is rotating at more than a thousand miles an hour, yet I do not spin off into space! With all of the pressure I put on it, my ass is now 8 percent denim.

Bottom line, pending extinction by meteor, suicide bomb, or greenhouse effect, I need to take better care of myself if I'm gonna outlive my genetics. Pharmaceuticals, diet, moral and physical hygiene—some things will help more than others. Most people who go on diets fail to take off significant poundage, and I'm probably doomed to be one of them. Even if I weren't, 95 percent of dieters who *do* lose weight put it back on soon enough.

Told that cigarettes were toxic, Americans began to quit smoking them, but controlling our eating habits has been tougher. We've tried the cabbage soup, grapefruit, caveman, wild salmon, fen-phen, pasta-chocolate, Russian Air Force, Mayo Clinic, South Beach, Slim Fast, Three Hour, Subway, Scarsdale, Zone, Pritikin, Atkins, Weil, Ornish, Jenny Craig, Adele Puhn, Gwen Shamblin, Crystal Meth, All You Can Eat, no-carb, Weight Down Workshop, and Weight Watchers diets, but 70 percent of us are still overweight. McDonalds and Wendys represent one end of the problem, while for those who can afford it, Charlie Trotter and Alice Waters feed our obsession with high-end cuisine. Whatever our budget, we've made eating a kind of religion. We want to *believe* with our taste buds.

In the face of all this, I have to lose twenty-five pounds and elevate my heart rate for fifty minutes at least every other day. I'd not only appear less ridiculous in a magenta Speedo (and a man in my position *cannot afford to be made to look ridiculous*) but reduce the level of lethal blubber bunging up my arteries. And I really hope the Zetia works, especially since I've heard about Niaspan's nastier side effects—hot flashes, impotence, permanent liver damage, fiery itches, and "flushing," which means your face stays bright red. (The joke is, you look like a hard-on but can no longer get one.) I'd still have no choice but to take it. I want to survive for the sake of my wife and daughters. When Grace is a freshman in high school I'll be sixty-three and a half, two years older than any McManus male in our line. With Niaspan, there I would be, limp-dicked and glowering like Mr. Johnson hisself, but on hand. Lucky Jim.

A few days ago Jennifer signed us up at a place called Lifetime Fitness, and as soon as I finish this book I'm gonna start swimming laps in their pool three or four evenings a week. (Hey, I'm serious.) I don't see myself as a candidate for a gastric bypass, despite their cachet among sedentary poker players, but I'm just about due for the other kind. I need to use old-fashioned will-power to stop killing myself with stemware and cutlery, though I'll take any help I can get from the doctors and scientists. We all would, I think. The smart folks in lab coats are saying that embryonic stem cell research is the best way for them to find cures for some of our most common diseases, so let's let them do their damn jobs.

I've also read about a magical drug they're developing to stimulate the melanocortin-4 receptor in the hypothalamus, thereby inhibiting appetite. If you take the right dose, your body sheds fat and gains muscle. I'll be able to sit at my desk or the dinner table, swallow a little white pill with a Newcastle Ale or the '01 Etude Heirloom Carneros pinot noir—which continues to provide delicate hints of rose petal before finishing with firm, chewy tannins—and thereby transubstantiate myself into one of those lean, ropy cowboys in the Marlboro ads. The most common side effect of MC4R stimulation suffered by test animals has been prolonged erections. So be it.

8 O'CLOCK SUNDAY MORNING

The people of God shouldn't be afraid of the people of science; we
need each other.

—BONO

동해물과 백두산이 마르고 닳도록
하느님이 보우하사 우리 나라만세 東海물과 白頭山이 마르고 닳도록
하느님이 保佑하사 우리 나라萬歲

n May 2005, as North Korea rattled its rickety but nuclear-
tipped saber, South Korean researchers accomplished something a bit more impressive: a new, improved way to synthesize
stem cells and transfer them to sick and injured patients. Once
again, it was the team led by our friends Dr. Shin Yong Moon
and Dr. Woo Suk Hwang. Their somatic cell nuclear transfer
technique was now refined enough to almost guarantee a personalized stem cell line for each new patient they work with. Less
than a year and a half ago, the team needed 248 donated eggs per
line; now it requires an average of 17. That number is likely to
dip even lower as the technicians growing the blastocysts and mi-
cromanipulating those fine-bore glass pipettes to extract the stem

cells continue to get even better at their jobs—greener thumbs in the petri dish, steadier hands on the joystick.

The lab's quantum leaps in efficiency enabled the doctors to put skin cells (not sperm) from patients into unfertilized donor eggs from which the DNA had been removed, then to harvest cloned stem cells that were exact genetic matches for nine of eleven patients, including a ten-year-old boy with a spinal cord injury and a six-year-old girl with diabetes. Personalized genetic material, of course, is much less likely to be rejected by the patient's immune system. As Gina Kolata reported in the *Times*, "It did not matter whether the patient whose cells were being cloned was young or middle-aged, male or female, sick or well—the process worked."

Many further steps must be taken before these patients, along with hundreds of millions of others, will be cured. Researchers still need to learn, for example, how to program the stem cells to grow into the appropriate replacement tissue. But doctors around the world agreed that the new South Korean techniques had advanced this hopeful process dramatically. The techniques will also help scientists learn how and why some diseases occur, which will aid them in developing drug treatments to interrupt the process.

Dr. Gerald Schatten, an American researcher who helped the Koreans—whose English is limited—publish their findings in the online edition of *Science* (www.sciencemag.org) on May 19, offered some insight into why they've succeeded when so many programs have failed. "They work 365 days a year except for leap year, when they work 366 days. They have lab meetings at 6:30 every morning except Sunday, when they have them at 8."

Dr. Miodrag Stojkovic and his team at Newcastle University are also making progress. On May 20, they announced that they had "created a cluster of human cells, known as a blastocyst, by inserting DNA into an unfertilised human egg and inducing it to multiply." The announcement emphasized that the team uses "unfertilised eggs left over from IVF treatment, with the consent of the donors." The researchers have thus far not matched the cells with individual patients, however. No word on when *their* Sunday meetings begin.

Even before these announcements, 72 percent of Americans approved of therapeutic medical research involving somatic cell nuclear transfer, as long as no cloned babies would result. On May 23 the House of Representatives voted 238 to 194 to repeal President Bush's restrictions on federal funding of research on embryos discarded by fertility clinics after August 2001. (The previous lines had been contaminated, after all.) Before the vote, Republican Christopher Shays said, "I think it's time we recognized the Dark Ages are over. Galileo and Copernicus have been proven right. The world is in fact round; the Earth does revolve around the sun. I believe God gave us intellect to differentiate between imprisoning dogma and sound ethical science, which is what we must do here today."

Even though forty-nine other Republicans voted in favor as well, support fell short of a veto-proof two-thirds majority. An identical Senate bill is being sponsored by Pennsylvania Republican Arlen Specter and Iowa Democrat Tom Harken, and supported by Republican majority leader Bill Frist. Senator Brownback, of course, promised a filibuster to keep the Senate from voting at all. President Bush vowed to veto the bill if it passed. Tom DeLay said, "We were all at one time embryos ourselves. So was Abraham. So was Muhammad. So was Jesus of Nazareth." So were Uday and Qusay, Saddam and Osama, and everyone's willing to dislodge a few skin cells from those biological entities. DeLay also neglected to mention the ghostly embryological status of zillions of ova and spermatazoa murdered by menstruating women and masturbating (or lovemaking) men every few seconds, though we were all at one time those things as well. As for the immaculately conceived Jesus of Nazareth, who's to say how, when, or even whether he became an embryo, let alone what he'd have to say about today's biomedical research? But this was a guy, we may recall, who was willing to painfully sacrifice his entire body for the benefit of imperfect humans.

As the debate in America continues, it seems worth repeating that clumps of undifferentiated cells outside the uterus, whether discharged in menstrual blood or cultured in a petri dish for therapeutic purposes, have no chance of becoming a person. Since they have no chance of becoming a person, let alone a copy of a person, it's misleading to speak of them as potential "cloned babies." To do so is either uninformed or politically cynical. We should think of them as blastocysts or, as the Korean team's paper in *Science* refers to them, "nuclear transfer constructs." Above all, we should note that the Koreans did not produce them by fertilizing human eggs. Rather, they removed the genetic material from donated, *un*fertilized eggs and replaced it with genetic material from the sick or injured patients themselves. The resulting clusters of cells will never be placed in a uterus. In about half the cases, no male genetic material was involved at all. They have not been "conceived," and no womb awaits them. The cells consist of human materials, but they are not potential human beings. The researchers strongly believe that cloning human beings is wrong, and they fully support their country's laws that prohibit it. The stem cells will remain in a petri dish for now. Their only destiny is to be programmed to grow into healthy spinal, pancreatic, or other sorts of replacement tissue, once the South Koreans or other scientists figure out how to do this.

The Greek word *blastos* means "germ" or "sprout." A cyst is an abnormal membrane or sac containing fluid. The cyst that sprouted inside Jennifer and ate her right ovary had several human characteristics—including hair, teeth, and cartilage—but could never have become her twin sister or any other person; it could only have killed her. It shared countless genetic characteristics with biological entities absorbed by tampons, as well as those that became our two daughters. No one has difficulty telling these sorts of things apart, though at some early stage they were virtually identical.

As the medical technology brought to bear at both ends of life becomes more and more potent, we need to look hard—often through electron microscopes, those offshoots of William Worrall Mayo's deep insight—at where we redraw the fine lines, and to guard against inhuman abuses. But to morally equate a wombless blastocyst synthesized solely to help injured and sick people with an embryo thriving inside a mother-to-be does violence to human language and spirit.

Woo Suk Hwang put it this way: "On the one hand, you have fifteen micrometers of skin cells, on the other a patient who has suffered from an incurable disease. Maybe this fifteen micrometers of skin cells can relieve and save the life of a human being next to me, someone who has suffered for fifty years or must suffer for fifty years. Of the two, which do you think is ethically reasonable to save?"

However we answer this question, the life-affirming research will continue in South Korea, the United Kingdom, and elsewhere. Dr. Hwang, for one, has a real sense of urgency, something that Bridget and millions of others must surely appreciate. "I hope we can apply these wonderful technologies, not only for my generation," he said, "but also for my mother's generation." The South Korean government has boosted the budget for his team of forty-five researchers and technicians by 50 percent, to $3 million. It will soon break ground on a six-story building to house the next phases of research. Dr. Hwang, it should be emphasized, has no financial interest in the techniques he has pioneered. "I want this technology applied to the whole of mankind," he stated, noting that the South Korean government owns all the patents but wants to share the information, not hoard it. It will soon open an international stem cell bank in Seoul to help facilitate research in labs around the planet.

In the meantime, I believe that our president, the House majority leader, and their fellow conservative Christian politicians are smothering American science while imposing their personal religious beliefs on the future health of all of our citizens. Any "culture of life," as they call it, that values clumps of wombless cells more than fully grown mothers' sons patrolling Iraq in cheaply armored Humvees, ignores the defenseless multitudes of Darfur, supports capital punishment, accepts collateral casualties in avoidable warfare, and seeks to quash medical research that most citizens favor but is content to leave tens of millions of them without health insurance, has a bottom line that can hardly be called life-affirming. It may even be called sacrilegious.

I also sense that when the stem cell cures come online, nearly every human being will cheer. When we're paralyzed by an injury or struck with a debilitating or fatal illness, we will feel blessed to have this technique brought to bear on our body. Even Dr. Kass will admit, "I was an early critic of SCNT because I thought it would lead to cloned children. Once you get the embryos—er, blastocysts—in the laboratory, you have all kinds of dilemmas about what to do with them, and I was aware of that problem. But on the question of therapeutic cloning, now that all these wonderful cures have been found, I changed my mind." Let's hope so, at least.

Meanwhile, in the steady hands of the Christian Dr. Moon, the Buddhist Dr. Hwang, the relatively late-sleeping Dr. Stojkovic, the modest but well-funded Dr. Lu Guangxiu, the Beth Israel Medical Center's Dr. Mehboob A. Hussain, and colleagues of every other spiritual stripe, the scientific method is moving things forward for all of us.

ACKNOWLEDGMENTS

Jonathan Galassi and Sloan Harris made this book happen. I also depended on the help and encouragement of Katharine Cluverius at ICM; Jeff Seroy, Sarita Varma, Spenser Lee, Susan Mitchell, Anne Nolan, Gretchen Achilles, and Annie Wedekind at FSG; Lewis Lapham, Ann Kyle Gollin, and Ben Metcalf at *Harper's*; Brendan Vaughan, David Granger, and Tom Colligan at *Esquire*; Heidi Julavits at *The Believer*; Steve Perrine and Tom Foster at *Best Life*; Dick Babcock and Geoff Johnson at *Chicago*; Paul Ashley, David Kerns, Mary Ellen McManus, Fred Novy, and Scott Turow.